Blink

Life After Locked-in Syndrome

By David and Sandy Nette

Published by New Generation Publishing in 2013

Copyright © David E. Nette & Sandy Nette 2013

First Edition

The author asserts the moral right under the Copyright, Designs and Patents Act 1988 to be identified as the author of this work.

All Rights reserved. No part of this publication may be reproduced, stored in a retrieval system or transmitted, in any form or by any means without the prior consent of the author, nor be otherwise circulated in any form of binding or cover other than that which it is published and without a similar condition being imposed on the subsequent purchaser.

www.newgeneration-publishing.com

New Generation **Publishing**

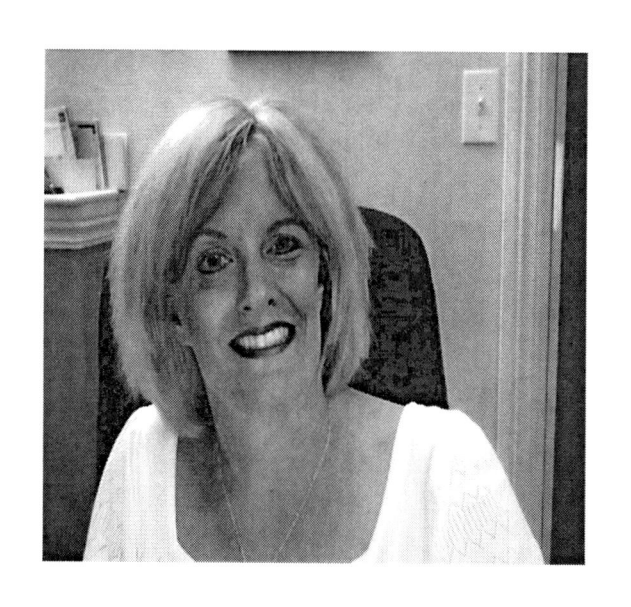

BEFORE STROKE; LIFE WAS GOOD

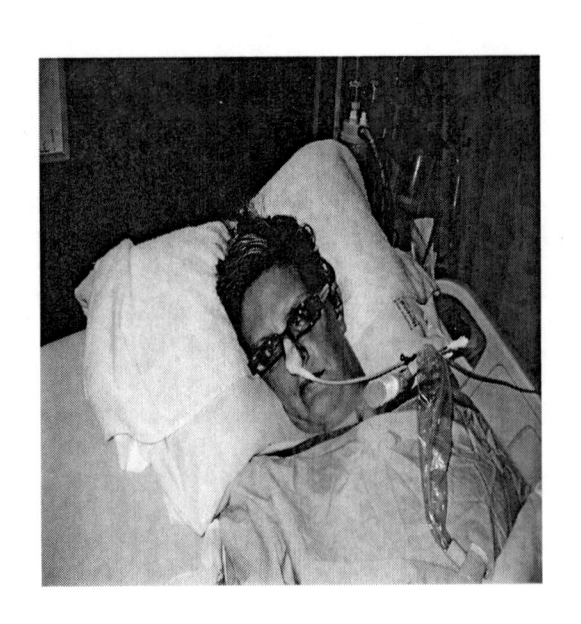

AFTER STROKE; FOREVER CHANGED

Blink
Life After Locked-in Syndrome

What Others Are Saying About This Book...

This is a story that everyone needs to read. It is a cautionary tale, a motivational story of trials, courage and triumphs but mostly it is a love story. An inspiring love story about a man and a woman whose commitment and love for each other serves as a touchstone and example for our own relationships.

Terry & Joanne Pithers "Style for Success"

❦

David's love for his wife, and Sandy's love for her husband, is the glue that has cemented their relationship and kept them going through adversity and tragedy. Reading this book will show you how, like a snow roller that leaves behind the imprint of its journey in the snow; so has Sandy left her imprint of courage, strength, determination and love on the hearts of those she met along her journey to a new and uncertain destiny.

Elizabeth Ohrn

❦

Sandra and David Nette's life was disastrously changed by a chiropractor's unnecessary neck manipulation. Unfortunately, they are not alone. In researching our book "Spin Doctors" we spoke with victims and neurologists who confirmed to us that many lives, like the Nette's have been destroyed, degraded or cut short by chiropractors who adjust the upper neck for reasons that are more religious and doctrinaire than scientific. In fact, there's no science at all to back up the common practise, it is a senseless waste.

Our meeting with David Nette, via a video Skype call, was one of the most difficult and heartbreaking interviews either of us have ever conducted.

The naked emotion, honesty and anguish was raw and unvarnished. He became a hero to us as did Sandy, who has suffered and risen above a cruel twist of fate.

The Nette's story sparks compassion, anger and faith in the enduring power of love. We're glad David has chosen to share it in his own words.

Wayne MacPhail and Paul Benedetti

❧

It's a WONDERFUL story of the power of love and forgiveness and how they can enrich our lives and bring us contentment and serenity. We all face challenges at various times in our lives - it's how we respond to them that shows who we are as persons..... You are both my HEROES!!!

P. Daryl Wilson, Q.C.

❧

My wife and I met Sandy and Dave purely by chance-- or so it seemed at the time.

Marge suggested that it was time to go somewhere other than Puerto Vallarta for our annual getaway from the cold. Being a creature of habit, I was more than a little hesitant. Not one to easily give up on an idea, she diligently shopped the internet until she found a great travel deal to Huatulco where we were introduced to and ultimately became friends with Dave and Sandy.

Although we lived in different cities we were still able to get together on a regular basis and the friendship grew.

One day, we received a phone call from Dave informing us that Sandy had suffered a number of strokes and was in ICU. The doctors didn't know if she would survive. We asked if we could come to Edmonton and provide whatever support was needed. Dave said it would be better if we waited until the doctors knew more about Sandy's prognosis. Two weeks later, Dave called and said that Sandy was going to survive and that we could come for a visit over the weekend. Those were a long two weeks for Marge and myself.

Upon our arrival at the hospital, I was shocked. Here was a once vibrant, energetic woman who now could only blink her eyes to communicate. She was now reduced to blinking once for "yes" and twice for "no". At the end of the visit, I whispered in Sandy's ear "I believe you will get through this." I was rewarded with a single blink.

At each visit, we could see the remarkable progress Sandy was making. Sandy's attitude throughout her journey was remarkable. She refused to accept that things "can't" be done. It was all about "how" things were going to be done. She possessed a fierce determination that she was going to control the situation and the situation was not going to control her.

Michael & Marge Weevers

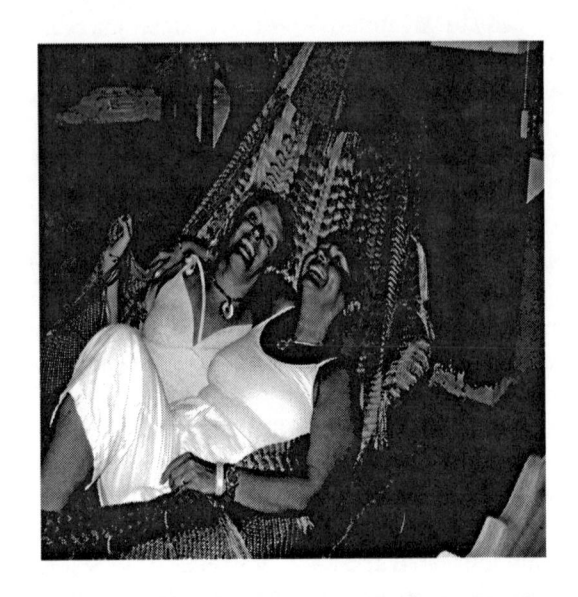

JUST HANGING OUT WITH MY FRIEND

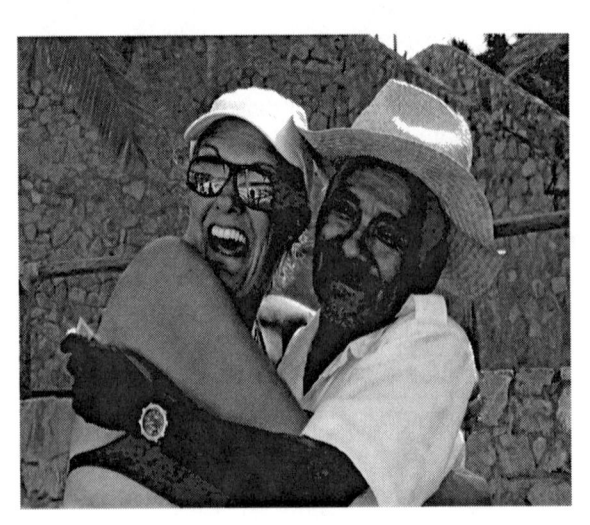

THE LOCALS ARE SO FRIENDLY

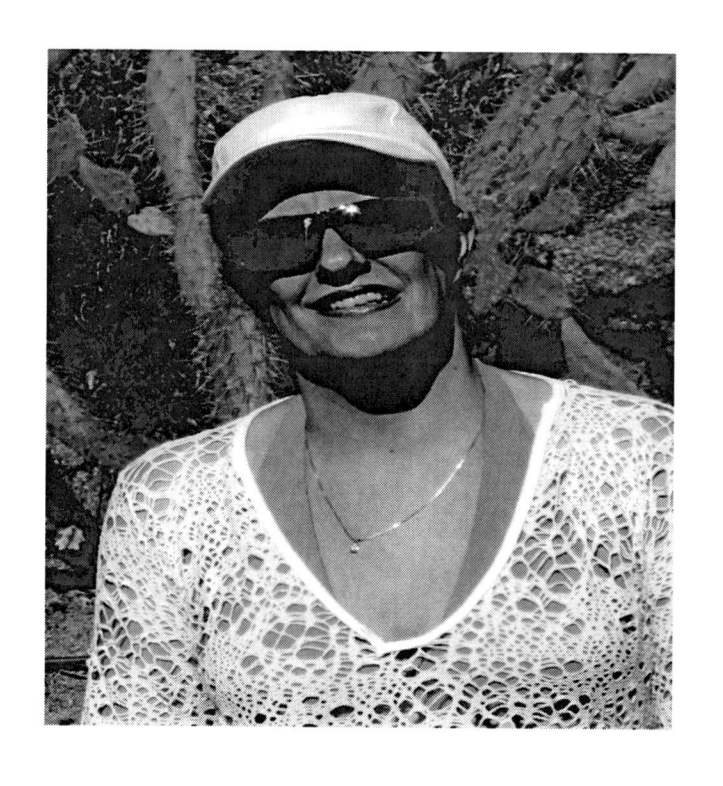

LOVE THE SUN!

Contents

Foreword by Dr John William Kinsinger...... 15

Chapter 1 The Beginning of Our Nightmare. 19

Chapter 2 Locked-in Syndrome 26

Chapter 3 Life on the Neuro Ward................ 39

Chapter 4 The Hug... 58

Chapter 5 Baby Steps 63

Chapter 6 A Brighter Day 75

Chapter 7 The Escape.................................... 83

Chapter 8 Rehab... 91

Chapter 9 Million Dollar Baby.................... 105

Chapter 10 Rebuilding Sandy 120

Chapter 11 Jaw Dropping............................. 134

Chapter 12 Forged Consent......................... 145

Chapter 13 The Freight Train...................... 151

Chapter 14 Moving Forward 155

Chapter 15 Sandy Gets the Last Word........ 159

Acknowledgements

To Sandy,

My reason for living life to the fullest; who, when most would have thrown in the towel long ago, showed tremendous courage and kept "moving" forward, one baby step at a time. Who was, and remains, the most caring, passionate and unselfish woman I have ever met. You make this world we share together a better place and I treasure every day because you are in it.

And to my loving and unselfish daughter, Linda, who makes me so proud to be a parent and sacrificed much of herself to make our journey a little more bearable! We love you Little Linda!

Many thanks to our legal dream team, Philip Tinkler and Daryl Wilson, from the law firm of Fraser Milner Casgrain LLP. Without their steadfast dedication and perseverance throughout this long journey, our future would have surely been made that much more difficult. We consider them amongst our dearest and best of friends. Thank you for never giving up!

We would like to thank Gareth and the team at Authoright.com who captured the spirit of our message and beautifully weaved the front cover into a powerful statement which could stand on its own. Your creative assistance with this project makes us very proud to be associated with such a professional organization and we look forward to future endeavours together.

And of course special thanks to the incredible Elizabeth Ohrn. Without her daily encouragement, editing and patience, this book would not have been possible for me to write. We thank you so much Liz!

Sandy and I are so fortunate to have the love and compassion of tremendous caregivers--both past and present! In our quest to avoid institutionalized care centers, finding good help is perhaps one of the most difficult things with which the sick and injured are challenged. Sandy and I often talked about this fact; and never took for granted what we had in place. For caregivers, it must always be more than just a job or they will never make it. Our caregivers were, and are, the best of the best and we vowed early on never to take them for granted.

Last, but certainly not least, Sandy and I wish to express our deepest appreciation to the myriad of nurses, doctors, therapists and other hospital personnel for all of the wonderful care she received during her hospital stays. We are lucky to live in a country where, despite one's lack of financial resources, everyone is entitled to receive outstanding levels of health care. Thank you for giving me back my wife!

Foreword
It Ought To Be A Crime

The act that caused Sandy Nette to suffer a stroke and one of its most devastating manifestations, locked-in syndrome, was no ordinary act of "malpractice". Rather, the chiropractor who changed Sandy's life performed his art exactly as it was intended to be performed. There is no doubt that healthy young people, mostly women ranging in age from twenty to forty-five, do on occasion suffer strokes following this procedure. The only thing not completely clear, is just how often strokes following chiropractic neck twisting happens. Some medical doctors believe it may be as often as one in twenty thousand; while many representing the chiropractic industry deny any link at all. Someone must not be telling the truth. In order to fully appreciate the significance of this issue, a brief lesson in history is in order.

Daniel David Palmer was an uneducated Canadian immigrant who settled in Davenport, Iowa towards the end of the nineteenth century. He toiled as a grocer and fishmonger; but he always had a strong interest in man's ailments, dabbling in such common day quackery as "magnetic healing". According to legend, it all changed in September of 1895 when Palmer cured a deaf man by manipulating, or adjusting, his twisted spine. Another miracle occurred shortly thereafter when he restored to health a man suffering from "heart trouble". At this point, Palmer was convinced that he had discovered the elusive single cause of all human illness, and simultaneously the cure. Palmer reasoned that the body was actually wholly capable of healing itself; in most cases the only thing preventing it from doing so, was a subtle spinal misalignment which he termed, the vertebral subluxation complex. Similar faulty thinking convinced him that he alone, had been endowed with a unique ability to not only identify these spinal aberrations, but also to accurately and specifically correct them using nothing more than his bare hands.

Palmer soon realized that this discovery was much too important not to be shared; so he opened the Palmer School of Chiropractic. Word spread quickly and Palmer trained dozens of eager young entrepreneurs, many of whom opened schools of their own. Years later, Palmer's son, B. J., advanced the concept that while the entire human spine was often afflicted by subluxations, the portion nearest the skull was of the greatest significance, and therefore, ought to receive the most focus.

More than a century later, D. D. Palmer's original concept of vertebral subluxation and its correction by adjustment, remains the bedrock of modern chiropractic; which in reality, more closely resembles a religion or a cult than it does a health care profession. That there is not a shred of evidence of the existence of such maladies is not of any real interest to the practitioners, their teachers, or the political bodies who have so deceived the public by granting them the title of "doctor". In the era of skyrocketing health care costs it is inconceivable that we could ignore the obvious fraud and waste associated with chiropractic, but it takes on a much greater significance when the voices of the dead and severely injured begin to be heard.

Sandy Nette is not the first, and unfortunately she won't be the last to suffer a stroke after having an upper neck manipulation. The mainstream medical literature is littered with the evidence of thousands of unfortunate young patients in North America alone, who have suffered profound, permanent injury or death following the manipulation of their neck. The earliest documented death from neck adjustment was published in the prestigious New England Journal of Medicine in 1934. Despite this ever growing body of scientific evidence, and a significant increase in public awareness, the chiropractic industry has effectively circled the wagons, denying their role in these senseless tragedies. If chiropractic neck manipulation were a drug, the authorities would have banned it decades ago. Unfortunately there is no FDA equivalent for chiropractic; it is a largely self-regulated industry, the classic case of the fox guarding the henhouse.

Not only is chiropractic neck adjustment dangerous, it is for the most part essentially useless. Chiropractors utilize neck twisting as more or less a "cure all", or panacea, treating everything from menstrual cramps to asthma. Conventional medicine is often associated with significant risk to be sure, but each decision to undergo treatment is balanced by the consideration of the potential benefit. Only when it is felt by both the informed patient as well as the physician, that the known benefits outweigh the potential risks, that a particular therapy is undertaken. On this count alone, neck manipulation ought to be outlawed as a nonexistent benefit, that can never be considered to be worth the risk of something as devastating as stroke, regardless of the rarity, if indeed it is rare at all, of such an event.

Sandy's tragedy, like so many others, is made all the worse by the reality that the chiropractic leadership has not only denied responsibility, but has actually chosen a "blame the victim" strategy in the effort to deflect attention from the dark secret that they have protected for so many years. It is long past time for the light of justice to shine, not just for Sandy Nette, but for the thousands of victims and their families who have, and continue to suffer, these senseless strokes.

The remarkable progress that Sandy continues to make is a testament to her character and her determination. In addition, the love and caring from her family and friends have no doubt given her the strength and motivation to press on in the face of impossible odds. In that regard, the undying devotion of Sandy's husband, Dave, is an example to be heralded by all. He has stood by her without fail through all of the small victories as well as the never ending setbacks.

It is time for Sandy's and Dave's story to be told; it is time, once and for all, to stop the madness that is chiropractic neck adjustment.

JOHN WILLIAM KINSINGER, MD IS AN ANESTHESIOLOGIST AND A PAST PRESIDENT OF THE OKLAHOMA SOCIETY OF ANESTHESIOLOGISTS

Chapter One

The Beginning of Our Nightmare

September 13, 2007

What a beautiful day. It was about 7:30 a.m. and Sandy woke me up telling me she had a great sleep. I stumbled downstairs which was my usual morning routine and put on a pot of coffee. I did a little pre office work while it was brewing. I went upstairs and took my wife her morning hazelnut flavoured coffee. At 8:30 a.m. a quick kiss and I was off to work.

At 10:55 a.m. the phone rang; it was my wife, Sandy. She told me she had decided to go for a chiropractic treatment, which was something she did on a regular basis. I was at my furniture refinishing shop which was very close to where she was heading. Just maintenance she would tell me, "Got to keep this great body in shape!"

Apparently she was about twenty minutes away and wanted to know if we could connect for lunch. The restaurant's outdoor patios were our favourite, especially at this time of the year.

I enquired about her exact location. I wanted to calculate if I would have enough time to deliver a surprise for her while she was out; something I had been trying to do for some time. No problem. She understood when I told her I was very busy; saying she would look forward to our time together later.

Perfect, I thought to myself. Without her knowing, I had the opportunity to zip home and deliver the newly refinished antique vanity, an early anniversary gift.

Little did I realize that this decision to go to our home and make the delivery might well have been the difference between life and death for my sweet Sandy.

The previous night we had gone to the Marriott, one of our favourite spots, to enjoy dinner while gazing out their huge windows which frame the North Saskatchewan River, taking in the gorgeous fall colours of the valley. It was that very day when we both verbalized how we must slow down and take it a little easier. Work, although we were both successful, had seemingly engulfed us into a frenzied pace.

I remember commenting to Sandy that we simply must rethink our priorities. It was during this time together, that I politely asked Sandy to trip over any life support plugs, should my demise ever seem eminent. The last thing I ever wanted was to find myself staring up at the ceiling and drooling into my lap. After all, I was ten years her senior, and we all know that guys go first. Little would we know, that not even twenty four hours later, it would be the other way around and Sandy would find herself in this catastrophic scenario.

Within the hour I received my next call. It was Sandy. She sounded confused and desperate. She told me she had to pull over and could no longer see the road in front of her. It took a while, but she was able to describe to me where she was…a mere five minutes from where I was located. She added that she was very scared and didn't know what was happening to her.

Panicked, I raced to find her. As I approached her car I could see the worry on her face. Although not able to drive, Sandy was still able to talk, albeit slowly. I asked her if she could slide over the center console and position herself in the passenger seat. I jumped into the driver's seat and began questioning her as to exactly what it was she was experiencing. I desperately wanted to calm her down.

Sandy said she felt extremely dizzy and couldn't see properly. Everything was apparently just a blur. Sandy was strong, but very frightened.

At first I suggested she might just be experiencing some sort of low blood sugar issue. We tried calling her family doctor from her car; but his office indicated that he could not see her until 2:00 p.m.; therefore, we took option B and headed for the Royal Alexandra Hospital which was just a short drive away. It was at about this point that Sandy said she felt a tingling sensation in her bottom lip and that her finger was numb. It just didn't sound right.

Upon arriving in the emergency bay, I truly thought Sandy was able to walk on her own. Opening the car door, I was shocked when she simply fell into my arms. Quickly reacting I caught her. Fortunately, a bystander witnessed this and grabbed a wheelchair. We were still oblivious as to what was happening.

We made our way to the triage and once through the formalities, we were escorted into one of their many emergency cubicles. Once in the Emergency Department, the hospital staff must go through all of the possibilities while assessing the patient. The painful repetitious questions of who, what, where, when and why began.

Once we made it into the emergency room, Sandy began to feel increasingly nauseous and very nervous. She said she had the urge to hiccup or maybe even throw up. Just prior to this occurring, I remember Sandy asking a young intern if she was going to die. I remember thinking Sandy must be overreacting. I was to be proven wrong...very wrong.

Surprised by the question, the young doctor quickly reassured her with an affirming "no", but he had expressed his suspicions she might be experiencing stroke symptoms. Not even five minutes later there would be NO QUESTION; she was having a serious stroke. It was immediately after this comment that the severe choking started and she ultimately lost control of the back of her throat and was gasping for air. At Sandy's young age of forty, the last thing one thinks about is having a stroke but this is exactly what was occurring. Sandy was having multiple strokes.

The choking became increasingly violent. I quickly yanked the privacy curtain open and yelled for help! Then her big blue eyes rolled back into her head and she began shaking uncontrollably. This continued for what seemed an eternity while they rushed to wheel her into the MRI room. I stood there feeling so helpless and fear gripped my body. It looked like something out of a horror movie resembling someone being electrocuted or a scene from *The Exorcist*. All that came to mind, was that death was tightening its grip on Sandy.

Eventually, Sandy was quickly wheeled out of the MRI room and the head doctor was telling me, "We have done all we can do". Chilling words that haunt me to this day. Then looking down at his open file adding, "Chiropractic treatment…right?" The pieces were beginning to fit together and it was beginning to add up, though my mind was still in a fog. I couldn't believe what I was hearing.

Still in a state of shock and disbelief, I recall shouting, "What the heck do you mean, ALL YOU CAN DO??? Isn't this a major hospital? What are you talking about? Please save her!"

The doctor stared up through his rimmed glasses and assured me that they were not giving up on Sandy. As quickly as possible, they would prepare her for transport to an awaiting specialist team that was at that very moment being assembled for her arrival at her final destination, the University of Alberta Hospital.

Time was of the essence, and everything had to come together for the hope of any success. There would be no guarantees because much time had already been lost trying to figure out what was wrong with Sandy. Our window of opportunity to correct and stop the damage from these series of strokes was rapidly closing shut.

I will never forget the intubation team that prepared Sandy for the ambulance ride. Sandy now completely motionless, eyes rolled back and struggling for her every breath was gingerly lifted by the surrounding emergency medical staff and placed on the awaiting ambulance transportation stretcher.

She was also a bit of a health nut, always careful to eat only the very best of foods. Rounding off her picture of good health was the fact that she was a non-smoker and never engaged in any "recreational" drugs.

Even the doctors would later comment that because of her terrific health and the way she cared for herself over the years, these things certainly played a factor in her unbelievable recovery process. Always maintaining a perfect weight, Sandy was incredibly healthy in every respect.

I would later find out, that following our hastened departure, the emergency doctors and nurses who worked on Sandy apparently remained standing for a full minute or two with hands held around the table where she had lain. Each one was standing in complete silence as if paying respect for a life in serious peril. They had done their part…now it was up to fate.

∽♡∾

Sandy's Thoughts

Waiting for David to find me parked along the side of the road was the longest few minutes of my life. I knew something awful was happening to my body and felt completely out of control. I was shaking and felt so alone and vulnerable; however, I was glad to be off the busy freeway. The fear was terrifying and I felt myself drifting in and out of the awareness of my surroundings. Sitting there all alone in the silence, I could hear my heart pounding. Things were quickly becoming surreal; and I vividly remember the sensation of feeling as though the speed of everything including my watch was moving towards a standstill.

I remember my heart pounding and the sweat running down my face. I remember straining to see properly--all to no avail. I would look at the dashboard and then look just a few feet in front of my car. Thoughts of my suddenly going completely blind overcame me and put me into a deeper level of stress and anxiety.

My thought process was becoming increasingly sketchy at best; and I could not understand what was taking David so long to arrive. While waiting these few minutes, I called another family member expressing my need to have someone on the line with me. I did not want to be all alone. Then the spinning would start again, and I would find myself completely nauseated.

I will never forget the moment David showed up and pulled his van in front of my vehicle. It was frustrating because I was excited to see him; yet when he entered my car I could not properly verbalize my condition to him with any speed or clarity. I felt like I was being engulfed by some invisible force and that my life was in some sort of unstoppable peril.

I will forever be thankful that David insisted we go to a hospital emergency centre close by, rather than attempting the long drive to my family physician. It would have been the end.

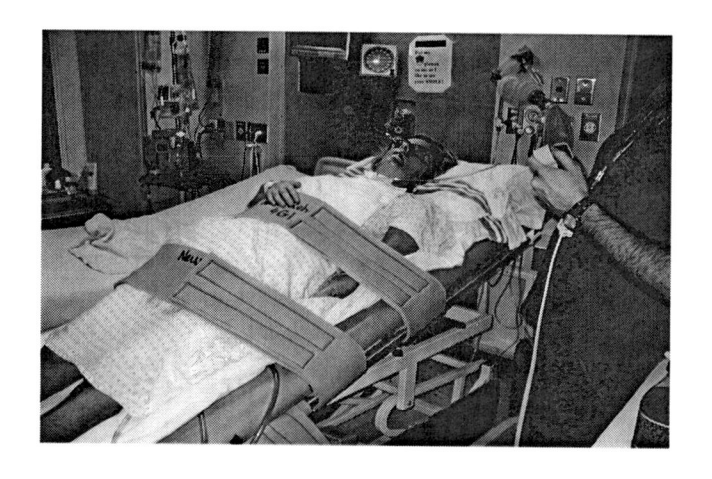

❧

THE TILT TABLE; OH TO BE ABLE TO STAND ON MY OWN

Chapter Two

༺༻

Locked-in Syndrome

For me, riding in the passenger seat of that ambulance, was the longest and slowest drive across town I had ever experienced. Time was standing still.

Looking back at Sandy in the rear of the ambulance, I felt like I must be dreaming. That this could not possibly be happening!

I wanted to throw the driver out and take over the wheel. Nothing was fast enough…or so it seemed. I felt so helpless; so out of control, so dependent on everyone else. It just didn't make sense; but as we approached the University of Alberta Hospital, my hope began to rise. Still I felt numb and anxious all at the same time.

Sandy was wheeled past the emergency desk and the nurses calmly asked for the paper work. I just about jumped out of my skin. Biting my lip, the driver exchanged a few words with her and we continued on.

Sandy was taken upstairs to where the Specialist Stroke Team was assembling. They were finished for the day and several had already gone home. Fortunately, despite being union workers, they returned.

The hours that followed were tortuously long. Word of her progress seemed to take eons. Then, while our friends and family members grew in number, the head of the neurology team appeared and updated me in a private side room.

The doctor, softly and as gently as he could explained to me that things were not good. Both of Sandy's vertebral arteries located in the back of her neck, had been severely damaged and that it had been a brain stem stroke--the most serious and complicated stroke possible. The risks were only beginning as he went on to ask me how far they should go if she happened to experience a heart attack or brain aneurysm while receiving the clot buster drip. This was a defining moment.

Our talk during yesterday's dinner was coming back to haunt me. "Well," I simply replied, "Sandy would never want to remain in a vegetative state as that would be no quality of life; but she is a fighter." I pleaded with the doctor to do all that they could; that Sandy would do all that she could, and we would leave the rest up to God. As the hours passed, our faith would severely be tested.

The numbers in the waiting area swelled to standing room only. Some commented that they had no idea that Sandy had so many friends–that they didn't even know that many people! Sandy indeed had more prayers going up to the Big Guy that night than anyone could imagine.

When Sandy was finally wheeled out from the emergency operating room, she was still not breathing on her own. They hurriedly wheeled her into the ICU.

When they let me go in, it was a very surreal moment. She lay there motionless, intubated but fully awake. She stared into my eyes. I carefully edged myself around all of the tubes and medical instruments and put my cheek next to hers only to feel a tear come rolling down. Sandy was not moving; but she was alive! For now that was all that mattered.

I called for a nurse to assist me with removing Sandy's contact lenses as I knew this was something that was always done at night. I would bring her eye glasses in the morning because without them she was pretty much incapable of seeing anything.

I spoke softly to Sandy asking her to please try to let me know she was okay. She blinked the one eye that was not bandaged. She was cross-eyed; therefore communicating in this manner was difficult. I asked her to hold her eyelid shut--which was something she could do. This was our first solid communication with each other since her cascading strokes, several in succession, and I knew I had my Sandy back! Confirmation at last! It was clear she was paralysed but she could hear, of that there was no doubt. And her mind was working just fine!

She told me through a series of yes and no blinks, one holding shut for yes and two rapid blinks for no, that she could feel everything! She felt every misplaced needle attempt, every cramp, the stream running down from her nose, her itchy scalp--everything. While this was great news it also brought with it the realization that she would have no way of scratching any itch, rolling over, stretching, or functioning with any independence. She was now at the mercy of twenty-four hour care.

As time would progress, we would come to appreciate the things that most of us take for granted--like the importance of being able to cough and swallow. This was going to be a long journey; but for now the goal was just to get Sandy out of the ICU and unto the ward. Sandy had joined the rare group of people in this world referred to as being trapped in something called locked-in syndrome--the closest thing to being buried alive. Some poor souls never do make it out of this captivity.

One day, one of Sandy's cousins, gave us a CD by Josh Groban entitled *Awake*. Such an appropriate title now that I think of it. It was early one morning and I was headed to see Sandy when I decided to slide the CD into the player. I didn't really feel like listening to music as I made my way back to the hospital; but the song called *Lullaby* started playing and I had no choice but to pull over.

Tears welled up as I listened to the words and it took me about fifteen minutes before I could regain my composure and once again resume driving. Like the song, the last thing I would do upon leaving Sandy's hospital room for the night was gently dry her tears. Many times her tears collected over the night and would form a small puddle against her face and by morning there was often quite the pool; consequently the need to place a soft diaper to catch the accumulation during the time I would not be with her throughout the long nights.

These incredible, intense and end of the day intimate moments spent together will forever be embedded deep into my soul. I will carry these to my dying day. It was during this time that my view of the world and life as I knew it would change... dramatically. It got to the point where I had to quit listening to the song for a while, as it was just too much to contain my emotions and people were beginning to wonder about me walking down the hospital corridors, at times sobbing buckets. Leaving Sandy's side was always the most painful time of the day.

One day while visiting Sandy at the hospital, I thought it might be helpful to place an iPod in her ears. With each of us sharing one of the ear inserts I carefully adjusted the volume and began to play one of our all-time favorite songs, *Over the Rainbow,* by our favourite Hawaiian singer, Israel Kamakawiwo'ole. The song didn't go over very well as it was just too much to bear for Sandy... and for me.

Although I was sad that I couldn't seem to break into her world of boredom and repetitive daily activities, I did eventually come to learn patience--even in this situation. I longed for something to give her joy. Her days of playing the piano were over; but I knew music was something she truly enjoyed. We would later come to try this again.

ورو

Loneliness

After spending sometimes up to eighteen hours a day by Sandy's bedside, there were indeed many long lonely walks back to the car each night; but at least there were no long line ups for the parkade pay booth. I stumbled along that path each night; the same direction so many times, that I'd swear I could have done it with my swollen eyes closed...then again, sometimes they were.

At the end of many long nights, I would often listen to *Lullaby* while wearing my iPod. The corridors take on a whole new feel during these odd hours. Many times by the end of the day, I would suffer from memory loss and found myself wandering aimlessly around the parkade looking for my vehicle.

Not a big deal; but when its -30° F and your eyes are flooded with tears, things can get somewhat uncomfortable. Once I even called Security to report my vehicle stolen! Truly as they say, 'of all the things I've lost, I miss my mind the most'. I did find a solution to this dilemma as Sandy's memory was perfect! Eventually I got with the plan; and upon my arrival each day to the hospital, I simply told her on which floor I was parked. She never got it wrong.

There are always moments that you remember, times that stand out and impressions that last a lifetime. For example, when I would come to the point along this walk through the hospital where the covered pedway led out to the parkade; it always struck me deeply to see all those abandoned, stranded wheelchairs--like discarded fragments of a path not chosen. Many had been tossed aside, not even coming close to their intended designated parking spot. Just like my little broken Sandy, some had their leg supports missing altogether, others had torn seats, ripped backs and were falling apart. The image just seemed to be saying something to me.

This was an eye opener. My view of life as a husband and the wedding vows I had taken became so real. For better or worse...how much worse could this get? I would go on to meet many others in the hospital struggling to find the inner strength to support their loved ones. Together many bonds were formed. Each and every person I met during this time, made me reassess my values and appreciate every day just that much more; and every day above ground is a good day!

༺༻

Helpless

No matter how much time I spent alone with Sandy in the hospital, I was always at a loss as to what exactly to say to others who were also struggling. It seemed we were always surrounded by people in similar grief stricken situations. Often providing a shoulder was all we had left. What do you say to a young husband and father of three toddlers who struggles to hold himself up against the wall when he is told by the surgeons that they really should pull the plug because his wife will no longer function as a normal human being? What do you say to a young mother who struggles with an infant son riddled with cancer or to be in the shoes of a wife whose husband just suffered a motorcycle accident and after three months in recovery still no longer recognizes her?

Adversity and tragedy have a way of bringing you to a complete surrender. In reaching out to the hurting souls and the injured, we both experienced every emotion possible. Thank goodness for our faith; as this would be all we had at times to carry us through. On a personal note, it was when I reached complete bottom that I finally got my act together and realized I was no longer in control of anything.

Day after day, this routine began to take its toll on Sandy and on me. I didn't want to admit it; but I was losing weight and was becoming a nervous wreck. I could no longer sleep and my appetite was dismal at best. I recall many nights lying in bed and wondering when my wife would return. What was she doing this very moment? Had she awoken despite her nighttime medications? Was she in pain? Could anyone hear her moans? Had the red alarm button once again fallen off her little hand? Was she choking or gasping for air? Were her lungs crying out for oxygen and her chest rising and falling at an alarming rate? Did someone inadvertently shut her hospital door….again?

Over the many coming nights I would not be able to sleep thinking about Sandy all alone in her hospital room. She had been transferred to a private room and while this had many benefits during the day; it brought with it much fear for the long and lonely nights.

One particular night, after spending sixteen hours by Sandy's side, I recall dragging my butt to our home computer. There I could sit down, gather my thoughts and find some familiarity - perhaps a fragment of some inner peace.

Going through our photos on line and looking at the many pictures of us as a couple enjoying the things we loved so much brought me a little comfort. I had visions of us on the beaches of the world, travelling together, spending time cooking and entertaining with our wonderful friends, canoeing, camping along the river or just spending time at our favorite restaurants.

Sitting there, I would garner what little strength I had left from the day and do my best to update family and friends on Sandy's progress. Writing emails on a regular basis became a way for me to release my frustration, anger and fears. It also kept people in the loop who, like me, were feeling so helpless. It also seemed like this was the right thing to do. I made a commitment to myself that I would share as much and as often as I could. I would share the good, the bad and yes, even the ugly.

For the most part, I kept this nightly routine for many months until one day I could write no more. Sandy had taken a step back and was admitted to the ICU. Her pulse was rapid and her breathing out of control. It quickly brought back so many desperate memories and feelings of extreme anxiety. Once again, she was falling apart before my eyes; and did not even have the strength to blink; therefore all communication was lost. After she was wheeled downstairs into the ICU, I stayed as long as they let me.

Once Sandy was all hooked up and I was assured that they would be watching her 24/7 I headed home.

I remember the night well. I truly had thought we were making progress. Sandy had regained some movement on one side and was able to squeeze my finger. Even the suctioning had gone down a little. Repeatedly I would ask myself how on earth this could be happening.

I was, sitting at my computer racking my brain for some word of encouragement I could pass along to my faithful "audience". Every time I reached for the keyboard, a wave of overwhelming sadness gripped me like a vise, stopping me in my tracks. I started sobbing and wept until I could cry no more. I pushed my chair back and crumpled to my knees. Then completely prostate, I just curled up into a ball and cried some more. My stomach tightened into knot after knot. I was like a child, completely broken and unable to walk.

Eventually, I did make it to the stairwell leading up to our main floor; but I was still not able to stand. I crawled like a baby on all fours. Thirty two stairs later, I made it to the bed, only to find myself unable or unwilling to even undress. I dragged myself onto the bed and under the covers. I tried to convince myself that tomorrow would be a better day.

As part of my usual nightly routine, I would place several phones on each side of my body. The hospital staff had all of my contact numbers. Then, as usual, I would lay awake for hours, sometimes getting as little as three hours of sleep a night. I would dream of dying and would wake up drenched in sweat. My fear was that Sandy would have no one to look after her; to be by her side or explain to the doctors the little things that were happening. We had had so many scares by this time, that I was feeling more and more pressure to oversee things; despite the fact that the nurses and doctors were all taking such good care of my Sandy. One day, a nurse asked me to follow her into a storage room full of files. She pointed to several rows of files which rose up from the floor to the ceiling. They were beginning to lean much like the Tower of Pisa. "Those," she informed me, "are the day to day records, tests, and progress reports for your wife. We are taking very good care of your wife." She made her point.

For the most part, the hospital experiences were quite good. Sandy's case was extreme and there were many unknowns. Often interns would enter in tow, eager to learn more of this strange and rare thing called locked–in syndrome. Both Sandy and I will never forget the day the lead doctor told the large group of interns to put their textbooks away. Sandy would now be labelled a tetraplegic and no longer would be considered to be trapped in this so called locked–in syndrome!

∽∽

Sandy's Thoughts

I remember waking up with my eyes transfixed on the ceiling. My mouth felt stretched around the plastic tubing which ran down my throat. My eyes were burning as they still had my contacts firmly embedded. I could hear various sounds from within the ICU recovery room but could not initially make out David's voice.

I was trapped. Unable to move or reach out for help; but still very much drugged from the arduous life-saving procedure where they had carefully managed to stop the blood flow from my ripped vertebral arteries. At this point, they had me at least stabilized and had stopped the damage from continuing; although all I could acknowledge was that I was still alive.

I remember David approaching my bed. Tears were streaming down his face and I can still feel his prickly face against my cheek. A few tubes would not get in his way!

He gently cupped his hands on each side of my face and told me that I was going to be all right. David said that we were going to make it and that he would do whatever needed to be done to get me home as soon as possible. Neither of us really understood the gravity of the injury at this point; but I was grateful for his determination and confidence--especially at that moment when I realized that I was completely paralyzed and unable to even take a single breath on my own.

David had asked me to blink and respond to his questions; but I really don't remember too much of these early recovery days. That first eleven days will remain for the most part a blur.

The following weeks would prove to be the test of my life. As the hospital gradually weaned me off the drugs, I became more acutely aware of my sudden misfortune. Over and over I would ask myself: "Would this be how I would spend the rest of my life? How long would I exist? Not live....exist. Would I even be able to stretch out and take a deep breath of fresh air again? Would I have some relief or devise a way of telling the nurses about my serious leg cramping? Would I have to endure my itchy scalp another minute without any means of getting assistance? Would I choke to death slowly and not be heard? Would I find myself actually looking forward to death? How long would friends and family continue to visit me because I was unable to even say, 'thanks for coming'?"

There are far too many things that I cannot share due to their personal nature; but I will say that very early on I became angry at my situation. I could handle many things; but I was always very independent. With a high pain threshold I rarely complained...unlike my hubby, David! When I lost all my privacy, dignity was not far behind.

There were conflicting prognoses by a number of tremendous and highly qualified doctors to try to comprehend. It was a real struggle, as we wanted true answers; but deep down only wanted to hear the positive.

At times I would hold in the tears just long enough for my visitors to leave and then Dave would get the entire brunt of my frustration.

I remember feeling very badly one day when a group of visitors all arrived at once. Unfortunately, although my hearing was and remains very good, for some reason I found it increasingly difficult whenever more than two people were talking at the same time. The room would seem to be reverberating. For this reason alone, we were forced to limit the number of people entering at the same time.

One day I remember studying the faces of those standing around my hospital bed. I had a private room by this point so that helped somewhat. I remember the silence. I had just come back from another near death experience in the ICU ward. These "friends" whom I had not seen in many years appeared in the room. I believe they had heard of my plight from reading the local papers. Dave had stepped out to use the washroom and was grabbing a bite downstairs.

It was so awkward. They were really shocked by my appearance and although I am sure they tried not to reveal their surprise, their horrified expressions said it all. The drool was running down my face and I remember being thankful that at least the feeder tube had been exchanged for a G-tube. Having that hose shoved down my nose wasn't a pretty accessory and made little in the way of a fashion statement.

They continued to stare and ask me detailed questions despite the fact that I could not speak. Then they would all just gaze with open expressions into my eyes once again as though expecting me to blurt out an answer. It was very strange. Eventually they must have conceded because they finally just all stood there and stared for what seemed like an eternity. One by one they left my room with heads bowed. It was like a death march.

Dave returned to find me pretty upset. I painfully went through a series of blinks and filled David in as to what exactly had happened while he was downstairs; but as usual we did end up chuckling when I could not tell him who they were. I recognized them as past acquaintances; but I truly didn't have a clue as to their identity. From that point forward, David would bring his lunch or dinner back to my room. He always worried way too much.

ชชช

Chapter Three

Life on the Neuro Ward

Initially, Sandy spent about two weeks in the ICU before stabilizing enough to be transferred to the stroke ward. During the next six months Sandy, as mentioned in the previous chapter, would relive this experience several times over.

As much as humanly possible, my days and nights were spent by her side. She was turned approximately every fifteen minutes and suctioned through her throat trachea. This constant need for suctioning (about every ten minutes) would go on for many months and was the main culprit for repeatedly sending Sandy back to the ICU.

It would be a full five months in the U of A Hospital before Sandy would free herself from the rubber hose that confined her to her room. It might as well have been a chain around her neck. There would be no chance of eventually going to the Glenrose Rehabilitation Centre unless they were successful in removing it. This meant Sandy being able to have a strong cough on her own. The changes in Sandy's condition during the next month would be the deciding factor.

Day in and day out, just lying in bed motionless, took its toll on Sandy's fragile body. It began to eat her up and she began to lose weight. At one point, I stood at the foot of her bed and lifted both of her ankles up a few inches and just stared at the flesh hanging down from her limbs. There was little if any muscle mass.

How in the world, I silently wondered, would she ever walk again, even if she could regain movement?

One thing at a time. At least Sandy had not completely lost her vision. I went home that night and hooked up the printer. After printing what I thought might help, I took the printout along with a roll of Scotch tape to the hospital. The following day, I posted my note above her hospital bed headboard. In large letters it read: ***Please Put My Glasses On Me; as I Want to See Your Smile!***

Hopefully this would serve as a reminder to all attending to her needs, that Sandy, although appearing lifeless and devoid of being able to communicate, still had her sense of humour and was fully able to hear and see providing she wore her glasses! At least, I thought to myself, we can help her to see the world around her. Prior to leaving home each day, I would call the head nurse, ask how Sandy was doing and if anyone had remembered to put her glasses on her. I'm certain that I drove the staff nuts.

༺༻

Personal Challenges

As for me, well let's just say things were a little rough. I could hardly imagine my memory getting worse than it already was; but the brain is a funny thing. The things that were once important, like phone numbers and bank access passwords, all went blank. On more than one occasion, I would find myself unable to retrieve funds from an ATM machine. Oddly enough, the strange world of modern medicine, and terms like glycopyrrolate and the mentioning of occipital lobe damage, became common. The stress was taking its toll. For example, it would be only a matter of time before I also would require medication to help with sleep.

One day while sitting in Sandy's room, a nurse came in and caught me holding my arms tightly across my chest and crouching forward. I was experiencing a trace of chest pain but wanted to remain invisible. The head nurse insisted that she hook me up then and there, to a portable machine. "Ever have high blood pressure Dave?" she asked. I shook my head. "Well you do now!"

The next day I made a doctor's appointment and from that point forward, I started taking a little better care of my health. Enough about me...we had bigger problems with which to contend!

As you can imagine, the long stay in the hospital had its challenges for Sandy. When I initially left Sandy that first night, I returned in the morning to find, stuck and dried in place, the soft washcloth I had placed on her forehead just before leaving the night before. The message was clear. The hospital would keep her alive; but *we* would have to provide the extras for Sandy. In the months that followed, the nurses and doctors would come to know me as a very familiar face. On average, I would be there sixteen to eighteen hours a day. Eventually I would no longer be able to work; but that's another story.

As with previous nights, I would wait for the evening medications to take effect; then, I would dry my wife's tears and cradle her in my arms until she slumbered off into an uneasy sleep. I would often sit back down and wait in the darkness appreciating the moments of peace to which Sandy was escaping for a few precious hours; where she would find comfort and once again be able to experience the true joy of living if only in her dreams.

Then it was my turn to apprise the night shift nurses of my departure and to give them the heads up on Sandy's status.

Time to Regroup

Saturday, September 29, 2007. I was rushing around the house trying to get myself together after just a few hours' sleep. There is always a sense of urgency to return to the hospital.

There was coolness in the fall air, and I could smell the strong distinct scent of decaying leaves; a smell on which Sandy and I had always remarked when walking along our river trails.

I felt torn, but knew that the nurses were right about my own stress level; so I decided to take an hour for myself. I needed a walk and headed to the very place where I had proposed to Sandy eight years ago. There was no one else around. It was early and perhaps a little chilly; but I appreciated the solitude. It was one of those surreal moments when I approached the exact spot and saw a bench where the old picnic table once stood. There were names inscribed on a plate indicating this was a memorial for someone much loved.

At first I felt this was not right; that somehow we owned this little piece of real estate. How could I correlate this moment when I got down on my knee and proposed to Sandy, with this spot now being shared? I walked over to the trail, took one more look back at the bench and just hung my head. Walking slowly, I began to sob. I remembered the hysteria when I tugged at her arm and reassured her that this was "our" table. I remembered the happiness filling her beautiful big blue eyes and the joy we shared that moment in time.

I suddenly heard footsteps in the distance and lifted my head. Approaching me was an elderly couple and I wondered if they had heard me crying. Should I fade off the trail or would this cause them to worry? Perhaps they'd think that I was some weirdo wandering the trails at the crack of dawn. I didn't want to frighten them, so I figured if I stepped off the path and pretended not to see them, they just might detour and take one of the many forks in the trail.

As they got closer, I could hear them softly talking to each other. At this point, my eyes were practically swollen shut from sobbing. I prayed they would not speak to me or make any contact while passing. I turned around and gazed at the flowing river trying to make myself as small as possible. Of course, as luck would have it, they stopped and said "Good morning young man. What brings you out here so early this fine morning?"

I collected myself, turned around, and saw that they were standing there, side by side, holding hands. I told them I was just reminiscing; sharing with them that this was the very spot I proposed to my wife who was now in hospital. Before I knew it, I was rambling on and on. So much for wanting to be alone!

Sandy had given me the best eight years of my life; and now the future was uncertain. This elderly couple shared with me that they, too, were dealing with a serious situation, although they didn't share what it was. Perhaps the wisdom they held from life's past battles of their own, they probably figured that I had enough on my plate. They expressed to me that their problems seemed pale in comparison to whatever it was that we were going through. I watched them as they walked away from me and continued down the path hand in hand. They were truly in love.

I went back to "our spot" and sat down on the bench. My heart was pounding and just then I had a ridiculous thought; what if I were to drop dead from a heart attack right now? It would make a powerful story for the local papers; but wouldn't that be a bummer? I pulled myself together, took some deep breaths and hustled to the hospital. It was time to go and see my Sandy.

Arriving at the hospital, it was apparent that Sandy was doing a little better. She was showing strength in her neck and could actually move it slightly on her own. She had done this once before, just a few days prior, but this seemed more deliberate. I wiped her nose and she pulled away to the side. I think she was showing off.

Her doctor stopped by and once again encouraged Sandy to do deep breathing. He was instructing Sandy about the importance of strengthening her lungs. Once stable, they would be able to remove her trachea. Unfortunately this was something she would have to endure for many months to come.

Trying to sweeten the pot, I told Sandy that once she could swallow again, and the trachea was removed, I would resume our morning coffee ritual and bring her any flavour she requested.

※

Red Flags

One morning, not long into this hospital stay, I walked in to find Sandy in distress. It wasn't hard to spot as her face was scrunched up and distorted. She was moaning, but of course unable to speak. She had heard me approaching from a long distance down the hall as I greeted the morning shift. I grabbed her glasses from the bedside table and quickly put them on her. I then ripped back the covers and attempted to see if there was a pin or something hurting her; perhaps it was the bed rail. Then I ran through a list of questions as rapidly as I could. Sandy...what is it, your head, your neck, a cramp, your stomach!!!!!! What???

I took out my pad and paper and we began the painfully slow process of communicating the only way we could. Sandy would close her eyes when I called out the correct letter. It spelled out as follows: "They told me I was going to die last night. I wanted to say goodbye to you. I could not see or respond to who was talking; but it was two nurses at the foot of my bed." With that, I rushed to the front desk and asked what on earth had happened last night! What was Sandy talking about?

The head nurse assured me that this could not have happened. I headed back to the room to continue comforting Sandy thinking maybe she just had a nightmare. As I was comforting her, the nurse came back and called me into the hallway explaining that she had found out what must have occurred. She went on to explain that two night nurses were apparently talking to each other in Sandy's room when they casually mentioned that this lady would not last through the night. THEY WERE TALKING ABOUT A LADY ACROSS THE HALL WHO DID PASS AWAY that very night. Needless to say, the nurses bought Sandy some flowers and this never happened again. My heart was torn in two thinking about what she must have experienced that night.

The months that followed had their ups and downs. We received great loving care from all of the staff; but the needs of someone in Sandy's condition were more than the hospital could provide. The nurses are overloaded these days and the doctors pressed for time.

Truly, this message needs to get out there, that when catastrophic injuries or illness occur, the need for family intervention must take place. The medical personnel can only do so much.

One day, just before leaving, I was told there would be another person sharing the already crowded room with my wife and an elderly woman. They were going to bring a drunken man and slide him between them. "Huh?" I said in complete disbelief! "Not on my watch!" And so it began...the standoff. Eventually after threatening legal action and citing safety concerns, (Sandy's air lines would be blocked from access to the evening respiratory team.) the person sitting downstairs that authorizes these transfers and placements backed off and apparently saw the light.

"Really", I thought, "my wife cannot move and you are going to put this guy within groping distance?" Perhaps taking the chair and blocking the door had some effect; I'm really not sure. I'm just glad I didn't have to get hauled off by security. I really needed to go home and get some sleep. I must have been going through sleep deprivation and was envisioning myself a hundred pounds heavier and one foot taller.

On another occasion, I walked through the door, and after just one look at her contorted face I knew that there was something terribly wrong. Once again, we would engage in the same routine, same rapid questions.

Pulling back the covers, I saw her right foot completely twisted around. It was turning a deep shade of blue, and did not look good. It was an honest mistake as the new nurse on duty did not realize when she turned Sandy, that there was a block of foam at the foot of the bed. This foam was to help prevent drop foot from occurring. This nurse actually turned out to be one of the best ever. She was a sweetheart!

It would be difficult, if not impossible, for anyone to understand the frustrations and the anxiety one would experience under these uncertain circumstances--being at the mercy of everyone around you; hating the invasion of privacy and the complete loss of dignity; yet also comprehending the fear of being alone and maybe choking to death.

Starving for air is a slow and gruesome experience. They were smart enough to give Sandy an emergency call button; but it would have been better had we been able to have one that worked! Sandy did not have the proper hand co-ordination necessary to press the darn thing; so in the beginning the call button was basically useless. Often the nurses would just take it off in the night because, eventually, it would just fall off and keep sounding false alarms driving them crazy. One can't really blame them.

At this point, friends and family all rallied around us, and it was reassuring to feel the bonds. The prayers and support of countless people was overwhelming. Despite this, it was extremely difficult for me to see my once strong wife losing hope during these early days. It was also sadly at this point, that some of the family members closest to Sandy began pulling away. Perhaps it was simply the fear of the unknown, or their inability to know what to do or say. Either way, it cut like a knife. When Sandy needed these people the most in her life and standing beside her, they were nowhere to be found.

Despite what Sandy described as feeling abandoned by her family, she also showed great compassion and forgiveness at this difficult crossroad. As the hours turned into days, and days turned into weeks, she had no choice but to either fade into a deeper depression or to let go of this part of her trials.

More than ever, Sandy was beginning to accept that moving forward, life was indeed going to be different and maybe if the prognosis was correct, even a tad shorter. She would take these lemons and make lemonade! She told me that she loved everyone and carried no bitterness. She added that she was determined to see the glass as half full, NOT half empty. Sandy was ready to surround herself with positive like-minded people and reach out to those in need.

Despite this determination, there would still be times of despair and moments of sadness. I struggled daily for words of encouragement but fear that for the most part they fell short. Although her mind was still sharp and she was fully aware of everything around her, Sandy could not respond. She became frustrated when I would jump to finish her thoughts. Sandy's frustration at not being able to communicate even the simplest of requests saddened her greatly. In Sandy's past chosen profession, she was a master of communication. Attention to detail was paramount and sometimes lives could end up depending on her decisions.

At this point in our journey, Sandy was too weak to even cry. She was completely trapped inside this almost lifeless shell of a body; realizing that she was fully dependent on all who surrounded her. I would help the nurses bathe her tomorrow.

Back home, I once again, found myself experiencing feelings of deep emotion. The house was so quiet. I recall walking over to the small antique vanity after the end of a very long day by Sandy's side and decided to fill up the small upper drawers.

Sandy had a multitude of perfumes and paraphernalia. I did not even know what much of it was, or what it was supposed to do. But this simple act seemed to bring me calm and brought me to a better place. Sandy would come home someday, I would repeatedly tell myself; and when that day would come, Sandy would rearrange everything and give me that famous bewildering "look" of hers. She would probably add, "Oh, you're such a man, David."

∽⋙⋘∾

Shake Rattle and Roll

I arrived at the hospital for what would be another long day. Sandy was struggling with the usual and I could sense a higher than normal stress level. Just by looking at Sandy's eyes, I could generally spot an issue in its infancy. Watching Sandy's chest rise and fall was another sure fire indicator; and of course, as the lungs would start filling with fluid, we knew it was time to suction.

I know for some of you reading this book, you may have a difficult time understanding or even believing what I am about to share. I will let you form your own unbiased opinion of the following account.

We were alone and I was about to call it a day. As mentioned earlier, this had been a rather tough day physically and emotionally for both of us.

I remember holding Sandy and bending over with my cheek resting against hers. I was praying out loud for Sandy, and holding her by the arms. I was praying for strength and healing; confessing that we were broken and losing hope; that we were beaten and had no more answers or even direction. Crying out for something to hang onto, I told God that no matter what happened, we would always trust in Him and never turn our backs on the faith that had previously helped carry us through so many other trials.

We prayed a long time that night; and something happened. Both Sandy and I felt an energy that was like nothing we had ever before experienced. Call it what you like, but that room came alive.

Sandy's bottom jaw began trembling. She had no control over this as the trembling became faster and faster and with more intensity. I kept praying; but when I heard Sandy's teeth start to chatter, I quickly stopped and asked her if she was experiencing any pain and if I should go get a doctor!

Sandy gave me a crooked smile and we used her letter board on which she typed... LOOK AT MY LEG! What took place over the next several hours would forever change my views on and belief in the power of prayer.

I ripped back the bed covers and almost expected to see some sort of problem or serious issue. I suppose it was just my low level of faith; but I was not prepared for what I saw. It was as plain as day. Her left leg had moved to the other side and was wedged against the bed rail. This was not how I had positioned it for the night. That wet, skinny, limp noodle of a leg, with absolutely no life in it, had moved over half the width of her bed. My heart was racing and I could hardly catch my breath. Thinking that this was perhaps something that had involuntarily occurred, I repositioned Sandy's leg beside the other one and asked her to try and move it again.

Sandy wiggled her toes and then as quick as a whip, moved her leg back to the bedside rail. I FREAKED! Tears flowed down my face and we continued to pray.

No sooner had I grasped the enormity of what was happening, when I looked up to see Sandy using her left arm to push against the mattress. This was terrific, as it would also help with her coughing ...an added bonus!

I took the left leg and held it in my hands. Pressing against the ball of her foot, I asked her if she could try and push against me. YES! There was movement and she was suddenly able to slightly resist the pressure against her leg. I could feel her pushing this "lifeless" leg against me. I wondered if there was anything happening in her right leg which had shown previous signs of movement. Sure enough, as I held her other leg up, just under her kneecap, she lifted her right leg straight out and held it up in the air for a few seconds. Over the hours that followed, Sandy also continued to show greater improvement in her right hand.

This turned out to be a VERY long night, as I did not want to leave Sandy's side for fear that I might miss another miracle. The nurses surely must have thought we were nuts, as there was a lot of shouting going on in Sandy's room that night.

I cannot speak for others, and of course we often do not understand why it appears that God is not listening at times. I do not understand why some must suffer and die prematurely. I do not understand why all of our prayers are not answered. We do, however, have a strong faith; and despite things looking very grim, we were at peace knowing that His will would be done and that we were not alone.

At best, both of us have always looked at life as being a short journey—just like sands in an hour glass. I thought to myself, that God must want Sandy to experience a few more rides. She is going to make it!

Anniversary in the Ward

November 2007

I called our dear friends, Derek and Kathy Stevens. They were there from the very beginning, even helping me the day I proposed to Sandy and asked for her hand in marriage. That was back in 1999 and it was a typical fall day, absolutely perfect in every way.

A quick call to Kathy and Derek, and Sandy would soon be in for the surprise of her life! I told Sandy the day was just too beautiful to be inside and suggested going for a walk in the park down by the river. The park is adjacent to the Storyland Valley Zoo in Edmonton. It's a beautiful peaceful place within the city and once you enter the park gates, it's as if you have been transformed into a rural setting.

All one had to do was simply stretch out one's arms with a little bit of birdseed and the Whiskey Jacks would land in your hands. Fall truly is our favourite time of year here in Alberta, and this day would be extra special. As we walked along the foot worn path, the leaves crunching beneath our feet and the river by our side, we came to an abrupt stop!

There nestled between the pines was a picnic table-- not just any wooden picnic table, but a lavish display of food, flowers and a wine bucket. As we approached the table out of curiosity, we could hear the sounds of Julio Iglesias playing softly in the background.

I remember gently tugging on Sandy's arm to get her to come closer to the table; but she was apprehensive and did not want to intrude on what might be the making of a movie production or some photographer's work. Of course, I knew this was all part of our plan, and although I could not see Derek or Kathy, I knew they would be hiding close behind the bushes watching to make sure that the wrong people did not sit down at the table.

Reluctantly, Sandy wandered slowly towards the feast. The bone china display featured many scrumptious delectables such as salmon lox, French bread, gourmet spreads, cream cheese, etc. The fresh white linen tablecloth was sprinkled with shiny decorations; it really was a sight to behold. I thought to myself, they nailed it this time! When Kathy said "leave it to me David"; she wasn't kidding!

By this time, Sandy was getting really nervous and just wanted to move on. She did as she always did when she gets nervous; she brought her hands up to her chest and started flapping. By this point, she was getting upset with me; but I forged ahead and sat down at the table leaving her about twenty feet behind me. I started by lifting the cellophane off the lox and sampling the food. Sandy scrambled for the bushes screaming that I was completely OUT OF MY MIND, as I watched the back of her heels running away from me. The gig was up. I had to come clean and tell her this was all a plan thought out well ahead of time. This was our table; I would tell her over and over gently taking her by the hand.

It took a little convincing before Sandy would agree to sit down and join me. I placed the linen napkin on her lap and filled her crystal wine glass. We toasted; now laughing hysterically, and just took it all in. After we finished our meal, and before packing anything, I knelt down beside her, opened the ring box and asked if I could love her for the rest of her life. Fortunately, Sandy said yes and there was never any need for me to even contemplate throwing myself into the fast flowing North Saskatchewan River, which was running close by. It turned out to be a wonderful day once again.

Fast forward with me now to November 21, 2007; our eighth anniversary. Despite Sandy's being in rough shape, as you can see from the picture enclosed in this book, I really wanted to mark the occasion in some way.

The nurses and doctors knew us well by this point, and agreed to give us some privacy in the room that evening.

In the early part of the evening, Sandy's cousin, Joel, along with his wife, Donita, came to her bedside. Joel has a strong voice and I asked him if he would sing a Josh Groban song. He had selected a powerful piece called *"You Raise Me Up"*. We were both so moved; even the thick doors in the hospital could not dampen the power of Joel's thundering voice as it echoed through the hallways. What a blessing it is to have such a wonderful family. They care so much.

Various family members would also come that night; but for the most part, we had asked for privacy. The day before, my brother's wife, Lorraine, had brought us an assortment of candles. We couldn't use real candles, but these were electric and flickered, creating a very nice atmosphere.

Later, Derek and Kathy arrived with a beautiful cake; and although Sandy could not eat any of it, it was a wonderful gesture and meant so much to us. Once again we were reminded of the kindness and generosity of our beautiful friends.

Looking back, although we would have rather passed on travelling this difficult journey, it has taught us many things; mostly how fortunate we are to have friends and family who care more than words could ever express.

If my little Sandy could have moved, she would have given the biggest hugs! If she could have spoken, she would have told them how much she loved all of them; but for now, they would have to read her eyes. Beyond the pain and suffering, was a genuine appreciation for the efforts of those around her. Sandy was not a complainer; and she would tell me many times over that "there was no time for the 'what ifs'; all we had was today, the present."

⊷⊶

Sandy's Thoughts

My recollections of the early days are somewhat hazy; but I will never forget the constant throat suctioning and the lack of subsequent sleep. What can I say? It was pretty gross. Visitors would leave the room, probably worried they were going to lose their cookies.

Eventually many of my regular visitors would just turn away and stay in the room while this brief procedure would take place. David was able to learn how this was done and actually preformed it quite well when the nurses were busy attending to other emergencies.

It would be many months before I would gather enough strength to be able to actually look at myself in a mirror. I relied on others doing a good job on my hair. I just could not bear the images of my deteriorating body. I looked as if I had aged twenty years over night. My skin literally began to sag everywhere, and my facial bones protruded outwards. My eyes sunk deep into the sockets and huge black bags formed underneath them from my lack of sleep. I was quite the sight; but David still said I was hot.

It's strange how life works and how it often teaches us lessons without our even realizing it. I remember many years ago when my father lay in his hospital bed dying from lymphoma. A nurse explained to us why he was not asking us how we were doing or what was going on in our lives, which had been Dad's typical style and his way of loving us and showing us how much he cared. I was about twenty one at the time and like most youth, my world was very small. The nurse gently explained that dad was in his last days and his world was now limited to the immediate surroundings around his bed. This was his time to get a little selfish; and to concentrate on just saying his goodbyes and hanging on to whatever dignity he had left. My dad was a tremendous father and provider, always putting others ahead of himself. Some struggled with his actions during these last days; but I can certainly understand more clearly now than ever, why this is often so common among those facing life's final chapter.

My father was a strong successful businessman; but he never stepped on anyone to get ahead. We were not rich but always had a wonderful home filled with the best of memories. He taught me many things that made me the person I am today. He taught all of us the true meaning of being successful. I know without a shadow of a doubt that he would have been by my side every chance he could, were he alive today.

I struggled every day just to survive. I could not really help David through his own trials although I was aware he was losing weight and looking quite stressed most of the time. His world was rotating around my circumstances. I wanted to tell him to just stay home for a few days and regroup; but I couldn't. I needed my husband more than I ever had before, and felt so helpless to return any strength or support. I determined in my mind that I would be there...eventually!

There would be times during this early period when my chest would feel as if a thousand pounds were resting on it--just like those commercials with the elephant sitting on the woman. My lungs took quite the beating, and despite the limbs beginning to show movement I was always reminded of how quickly things could deteriorate. I would continually use the little plastic blow tube 'toy' and practice deep breathing. The day I managed to move that little disk up a quarter of an inch was quite the accomplishment!

During these early days, I kept asking David when I would be able to go to the Glenrose for rehabilitation. Like a broken record, I would force David to get a pen and paper and write down my thoughts and questions. By this time I was getting a pretty good grip with my right finger and together we could motor along quite nicely through the alphabet. Little did I know that my husband was doing his best to get me off track and quit asking him. I later learned that he had had many discussions with various medical staff and David knew full well it was going to be many more months before I could make good my escape.

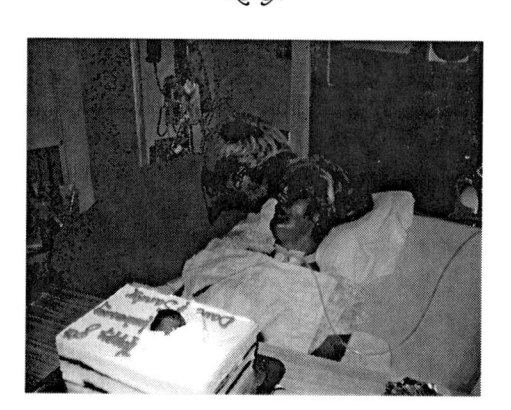

೩೨

I CANNOT EAT BUT IT SURE LOOKS GOOD

Chapter Four

༄༅

The Hug

As I write this book, it brings back such a mixture of emotions. Like anyone who experiences a catastrophic event and spends any time dealing with it on an ongoing basis it will leave its mark.

Memories are a good thing; but at times I must step away from writing and remind myself just how fortunate we all are. In the depths of despair one is provided with a means of measuring joy. For me, that defining moment was one lonely cold night, just before leaving Sandy's side. I leaned over to place my cheek next to hers and then we would do the butterfly kisses, eyelid to eyelid.

I got up and felt a surge of emotions and something made me turn and get just one more kiss in before leaving. As I once more put my arms around her shoulders and gave her a cuddle, I felt something touch and press into the lower small part of my back. It was Sandy! She was trying to hug me!! It had been so long since I had felt her reach out and touch me. At first I thought it was the night nurse trying to get my attention. I burst into tears and we sobbed together for what seemed like hours. Leaving Sandy alone that night in particular, and going home was very difficult.

༄༅

The ICU...AGAIN!

Sandy encountered some breathing issues right about this time and once again ended up being rushed into the ICU. These became such terrifying times of despair, realizing how precarious this tight wire walk was. Never really being able to let our guard down, Sandy's lungs were being worked to the limit. Over time, we lost count of the number of chest x-rays that were taken.

This time in particular, it did not look good. Her heart rate was racing, her breathing extremely laboured and she was turning blue. When they rushed Sandy downstairs I had to run just to keep up. They flushed her with frozen plasma and started suctioning aggressively. They felt she had caught pneumonia and once again, it would be the waiting game. They induced her with every powerful drug they had, even before the test results came back. Sandy was put into quarantine which really bothered her.

I thought, "How could this be happening?" I would come to find myself asking this question again and again. Sandy would get so far; and then have a major life threatening setback. I felt a heavy heart that night; but knowing she was being watched every second I felt that at least I could catch up on a little sleep.

I arrived early the next day and gowned up. They had Sandy sitting up in a Stryker bed behind the glass walls. My glasses were fogging up almost as soon as I entered the room. Wearing the mask always did this and I was tripping over the gown and shoe booties as I approached Sandy.

As the nurse on duty brought me up to date, I could not help but notice that Sandy was crying but she had a half crooked smile on her face! "What the heck was going on?" I thought; and "give me some of those drugs!"

It turns out that Sandy had a positive reaction to her spike in temperature and another miracle had happened. As a direct result, she could now feel movement in her jaw and the left side of her face. More importantly, she could feel her tongue rubbing against the inside of her cheeks! This was the only part of her body that previously had no real sensation. Even her speech volume seemed to be up! With that, the nurse opened the confining glass doors and took off her mask. She then cranked up the country music advising that I could do the same. Sandy had just turned it around in record time. ALL GOOD! I stripped out of the protective garments and hugged Sandy for a very long time! I still do not know why Sandy agreed to country music being played because she never really liked it before now. I was the cowboy. I thought maybe she was just back to herself and trying to be polite.

∽⌇∾

Battling Forward

Once back on the ward, Sandy would continue to surprise me. It seemed as if she would wait, almost deliberately, until it was very late in the evening; and then bingo! Another miracle would happen.

One night it was her toe. Yes, her toe moved! I ran out and grabbed the nurse, a large-statured young man and physically guided him into her room by his shoulders to see what I just witnessed. At a fevered pitch I encouraged my wife to show him what she had just accomplished only moments ago. "Wiggle your toe, again", I urged her!! "Show him!! Go ahead honey;

show Dean what you can do!" Seconds passed. Minutes crept by...nothing. Zippo.

Finally Dean had to go, but he said that he believed me. He gave Sandy the thumbs up and was on his way. Sandy loved to see me squirm. Perhaps it was part of her diabolical sense of control or a warped sense of humor. She was definitely a rascal at times and I would soon come to appreciate her funny tactics.

I recall one Tuesday night in particular, months later, when I would eventually take brief breaks and go for my weekly dinner at our friends' Derek's and Kathy's home. Sandy was being watched at the hospital by our dear friends and neighbors, Barry and Norma.

I barely got to my destination when I received a frantic call from Norma saying Sandy was having what they thought might be a heart attack. Apparently Sandy had spelled out the letters HEART; and then she pointed to her heart! That's all it took for Norma to burst into action. Next thing you know there was a code blue and a team running into Sandy's room with everything but the kitchen sink. Later she jokingly told me that she had gotten indigestion that night. Sandy said the attending team doctors were handsome. I could have just about croaked. Get your hugs in everyone and never put them off until tomorrow!

∽∽

Sandy's Thoughts

I really did have some fun...At times it was at David's expense; but I make no apologies. Those were tough days and I needed to occupy my time.

I liked reading this chapter. Despite the tough times in the ICU we really grew close as a couple during these months in particular. At times I laughed so hard I hurt my throat. I'm sure glad that David is a good sport and has such a wonderful sense of humour..

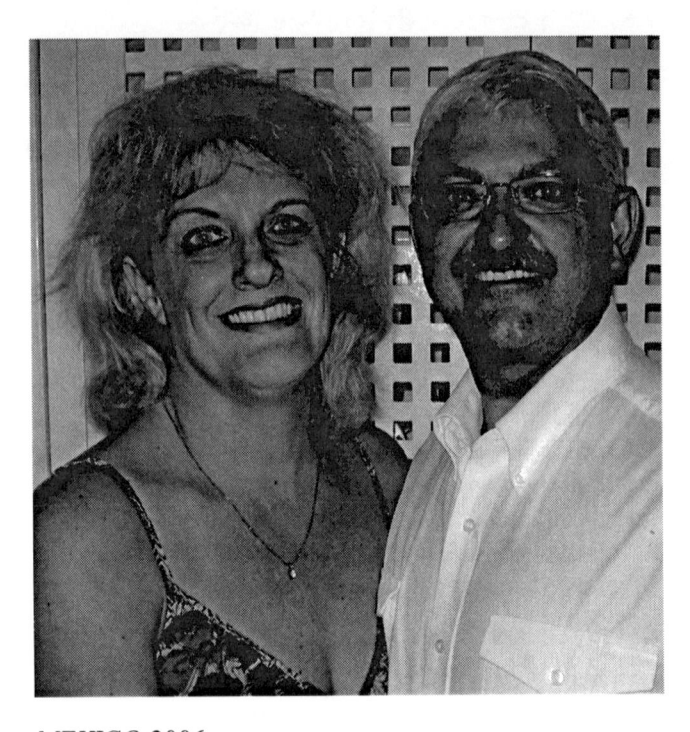

ಲ⋑ಲ

MEXICO 2006

Chapter Five

ଏହି

Baby Steps

Sandy was stressed out....again! Rather than giving her more drugs, a nurse suggested that I take off my shoes and lay beside Sandy. Hmm....sounded good to me; and amazingly this worked! After this, Sandy would need little else to calm her fears. It seems ridiculous, but this small thing changed so much for us. We thank the nurse who suggested this simple, yet highly effective experiment. Sometimes it's the little things that make a difference; while the obvious often goes unnoticed.

There were moments of humor; like the time Sandy and I noticed a fellow in a wheelchair speed past her open doorway. He was hard to miss as he was wearing a bright blue helmet and appeared to have long remnants of white cloth trailing behind him. Suddenly he did a backward flip and was airborne, his wheelchair landing on top of him. His gown wrapped around his head, and there was only moaning to be heard. Everyone came running to his aid. Apparently he had escaped from his secured bands once before. We called him The Great Houdini; and we were glad that he at least had head protection.

For the most part, things progressed painfully slowly; but things did move forward and eventually Sandy was allowed to come home for a day visit. It had been five months and the trachea, after several failed attempts to remove it, was finally out. Freedom at last! We packed her day supplies--feeding tubes, meds, etc. and waited for the limo, I mean the DATS bus to arrive.

The nurses accompanied us out that first time and shed some tears. We were a sappy bunch.

❧

Some Independence

The following week we asked for another reprieve from hospital life, figuring we could manage an entire weekend on our own. Oh, how we longed for privacy!

We opted to cab it this time and ordered a wheelchair accessible taxi van. The driver was so courteous, even putting on a video of Michael Jackson's *Thriller* for Sandy to enjoy on the long trip home.

At one point, I looked back to see Sandy enjoying herself. However, once Sandy was unloaded and we were in the house, Sandy asked me a question. She pointed to her letter board and spelled out: "Just how would you like to be stuck in the back of a cab for fifty-five minutes watching the credits continually run down the screen over and over again all the while listening to the thumping beats of *Thriller*?" She was unable to tell the driver that he had the CD on loop.

One of the things that I've noticed while writing this book, is that it's rather therapeutic. Part of me has been putting off this project. With the difficult memories there are also moments of joy and extreme jubilation; private moments, special moments and just remembering.

Spending almost one year in hospital care had its moments. While Sandy was in the hospital and in the little spare time that I had, the home renovations began. Despite being told that Sandy might never leave the hospital, let alone be transferred to the Glenrose Rehabilitation Centre, my goal never wavered to get Sandy back into her own home. This meant stretching the finances like they had never before been stretched. It was during this time that our family and friends extended compassion and helped us out financially.

It was also at this time that we discovered we had exceptional friends that we never even knew we had. Complete strangers opened their wallets and their hearts without having ever met us. Our faith in humanity grew by leaps and bounds.

༺༻

The Lonely

I am reminded of the many walks through the hospital's corridors, trying to wrap my head around what was happening. It didn't seem fair, so much suffering and so many lonely people. As I would leave Sandy's room in the evenings, for the most part I was lost in my own world just trying to make it through another day and get home to regroup.

Difficult as it was at times, I would glance into open rooms while walking slowly. I remember one young girl who always seemed to be sitting up in bed, rocking back and forth, tears often flowing, our eyes would typically meet. This is the brain recovery ward I would remind myself. But what was this girl thinking and what was tormenting her? I knew that my wife had all of her faculties and they were working just fine. I would think to myself, "Why was no one sitting with this young girl? Why was no one holding her, and comforting her in her time need? Where was her family? Did she have any sisters, any brothers, a mother or father?" My heart broke. After several months, we did manage a connection of sorts. So as not to encroach on any privacy, we would just exchange a warm smile. This would have to suffice and a friendly hello was always sent her way.

Though extremely limited in communication abilities, Sandy was able to make many friends in the hospital. I recall one day when the head nurse brought a young gal into her room. The girl was in a wheelchair and could not hear. She was being transferred to another facility. Forgive me, but I forget her name but never her big smile. We used to bring her candy on a regular basis and she would squeal with delight. Apparently she didn't have any visitors, either. It was a sad day to see her leave; but we were happy for her. The nurse turned her head away from us and cried. We were so grateful this nurse took the time to help send a little happiness her way.

※

Dirty Laundry

We have thought long and hard about how to share some of the serious issues along this journey. One of the most sensitive issues that certainly gave us the most emotional pain was caused by the actions or lack thereof, of a few close family members. The people we grew up with....the ones who constantly said, "If anything were to happen to you, I would always drop everything and be there for you." Unfortunately these much needed visitations would become something of a novelty and a rare exception. These times tested every ounce of our faith and inner strength.

For whatever the reason many injured or sick people probably have similar stories. Anyone, for that matter who has spent time recovering and has required a need for outside help can surely relate. It's so sad that these lessons are so painful; but they do strike at the very heart, hence the extreme sense of despair. We now believe that it was traveling through these stressful times in particular that caused the greatest inner growth. There truly can be a silver lining in every dark cloud. We just don't always recognise it at the time. As they say, a lump of coal must go through a heap of pressure before becoming valuable.

To try to take you into our world and let you experience what we were feeling, is not an easy task. Sandy's life was turned upside down. In the blink of an eye everything changed. By this point, she was dependant on the nurses turning her every twenty minutes and repositioning her body. She needed assistance with breathing. She could not scratch an itch, or if in the middle of the night were she to get a serious cramp, not only could she not relieve herself of such pain by simply rubbing out the knot but she could not even call out for help.

Looking back, I recall one afternoon which became a dramatic turning point where we would come to understand that this was going to be a long haul and we were in this on our own. Sandy had been in the hospital for a couple months and was awaiting the visit from a very close family member. This person had promised to be there by 3:00 p.m. that day. I was nearing exhaustion and welcomed the relief of someone else to sit by Sandy's side if only even for a few hours.

At about 2:45 I stepped out of the room briefly leaving Sandy and made a quick call asking about how close this visitor was to the hospital. "Sorry", came the casual reply," I'm still in Calgary at work and can't make it...something has come up". Completely stunned, I really didn't know what to make of this. I knew it would devastate Sandy. I politely ended the call saying I would try to console Sandy and left it at that.

As I opened the large door to her room, which now seemed heavier than ever, and looked down at Sandy whose eyes was still fixated on the clock, my eyes welled up with tears. I could barely speak and felt like someone just punched me in the gut. Sandy had literally been watching the clock hands for weeks, anticipating this special visit. Now my task was to try to convince Sandy that something very important must have come up for this important visit to not be happening.

Sandy was drooling and her face was completely contorted. I knew that she was wondering what could possibly be more important than spending a few hours together with this family member, especially when there was no guarantee of a tomorrow. These were the worst of times health wise, and every single day was torture. There are absolutely no words to describe what Sandy felt during this time. All I could do was gently take the soft washcloth by her bedside and wipe away her flowing tears. Cradling her body and pulling on the mattress cover I rotated her slowly to her other side…away from the menacing clock. She seemed numb, and other than the tears, I would not have felt her pain.

On the positive side, there were so many angels. People who were there every day to provide support in any way they could. Late night muffins would arrive at the door with Sandy's sweet Aunt Nadia. I think she really worried about me and just wanted to assist in keeping up my strength. She would sometimes chat; other times just sit and share tears, laughs or whatever the moment required. She was like clockwork.

Our cousins and friends were unbelievable. We are the luckiest people in the world to have such support and kindness. Everyone will go through trials at one point or another during his or her lifetime. And mark my words; you will be surprised just who steps up to the plate when the chips are down. Some, naturally with challenges of their own, might be restricted; but through cards and phone calls even those who were struggling themselves would reach out.

Complete strangers rushed in when it looked inevitable that we would lose our home. When Sandy needed a home gym, people jumped in to help. When our backs were breaking and we were having trouble lifting Sandy up our stairs in her wheelchair, the angels/neighbours were there to carry her up. One day I looked out the back patio door, and saw a whole crew of our friends preparing the outside deck for the elevator lift. Every time we turned around, we saw kindness; and our faith in humanity grew by leaps and bounds. We questioned how we would ever pay this forward.

On that note, installing the home gym was something that proved to be one of the best things that could ever have happened for Sandy. We were approaching the colder months of Alberta, and because of Sandy's complications with her lungs we were faced with having to cancel her local gym membership. It would not be worth taking the chance of her ending up in the ICU again. The last thing Sandy needed would be to catch a cold. Getting all sweaty in a gym and afterwards having her lungs hitting the cold air just couldn't happen.

The thought of Sandy's incredible progress taking a step backwards or her losing muscle mass she had worked so hard at attaining, was not an option either. We would have to find a way to make installing a workout gym within our home happen. The cost would be substantial; and at this point we were already worrying about how we were going to be able to hang on to our home. W5 had done a feature on us and we admitted on National TV that this event had all but crippled us financially. I think it was at this time that a few family members dropped out of sight. We couldn't really blame them!

Then right out of the blue, came more angels. Some incredibly generous and kind friends of ours, Irv and Dianne, dug into their personal pockets and made it happen for Sandy. Now, it would not be just any run of the mill gym but the best money could buy. There would be no more fears of Sandy having to stop her daily training regimen.

Specific weight lifting machines were installed that for the most part Sandy would be able to operate by herself, with no fears of weights falling or cables getting tangled in her hair! This, along with being able to purchase some specialized therapy exercise machines, Sandy would not miss much. And she was finally able to not have the weather dictate her progress.

Following a broadcast on CTV, we were equally stunned to find our mailbox stuffed with numerous cheques; mostly from people we didn't know--complete strangers wanting to do their part. It just seemed so unreal. At this point every spare dollar was going into the necessary preparations to get our Sandy home on a permanent basis!

It did not matter what the skeptics were saying. Each time they would enter the room and tell us we had to have a long term institution plan for Sandy; we always said things were in place and she would be coming back home. Although we had heard that Ponoka had the best rehabilitation facilities in the province for Sandy's situation, it was simply out of the question as this would have meant many days apart from each other. We had problems being away from each other for mere hours!

Sandy's Thoughts

Being able to go home and spend some hours alone with my husband was a turning point for me. It gave me the hope I needed at a low point in my long journey. It came at a time when I was deeply affected by the actions of a few. It's funny how we so often gravitate towards the bad things that are happening in our lives and how often we don't notice all of the positive things right in front of us. We have forged friendships that will last a lifetime. I have discovered a new me. ...the real me.

I will always remember Dave coming in the room with the young nurse and approaching the bed. When he took his shoes off and climbed in beside me I nearly fainted. I did not realize that she was in fact the instigator. I could have given her the biggest kiss!

Today, thankfully, we are finding creative ways to pay the kindness forward but my own life and my way of problem solving, has taken on new dimensions. In the past I was way too quick to express myself and didn't always use that much tact. Black was black and white was white. Today, I am noticing a lot of shades of grey!

I still have a long way to go as far as dealing with past hurts; but recognize that no one is perfect and we all make mistakes. What was, and is important for me, is finding understanding and accepting the differences creating common ground in order to move ahead.

Reading and working on this chapter with David was one of the toughest because it went right to my core. It's hard to believe, but these damaged relationships caused me as much or more pain than the injury itself. I am so happy that I can honestly say with all my heart, that I forgive and want only the best for everyone in this world we share together.

I'm glad to be moving on to Chapter Six; but must admit to having a good chuckle again remembering the past shenanigans of the Great Houdini. At times, it was better than a three ring circus on that ward!

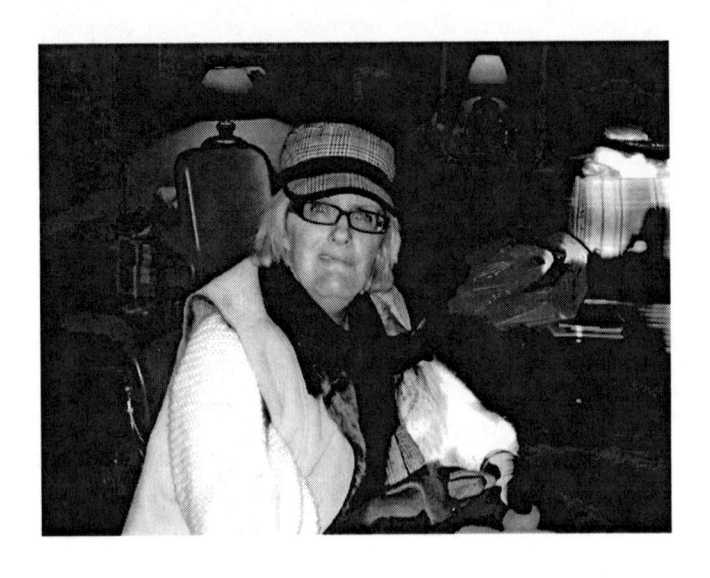

FIRST SHORT TRIP AWAY FROM THE HOSPITAL

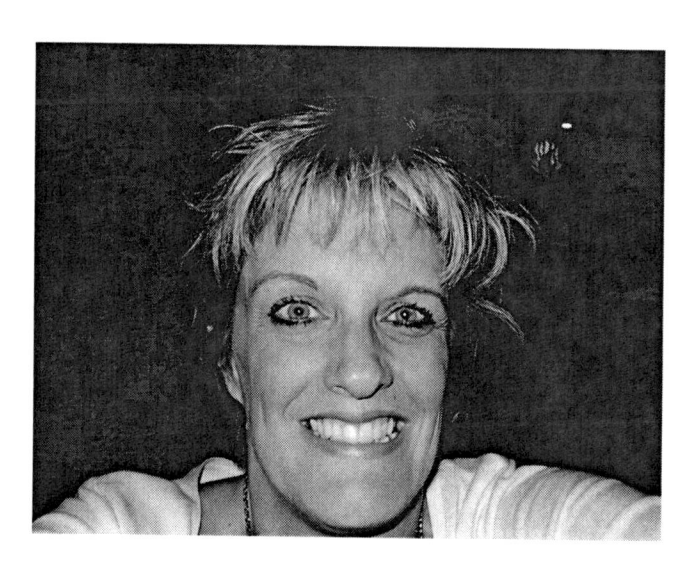

I CAN TAKE GOOD PICTURES OF MYSELF DAVE

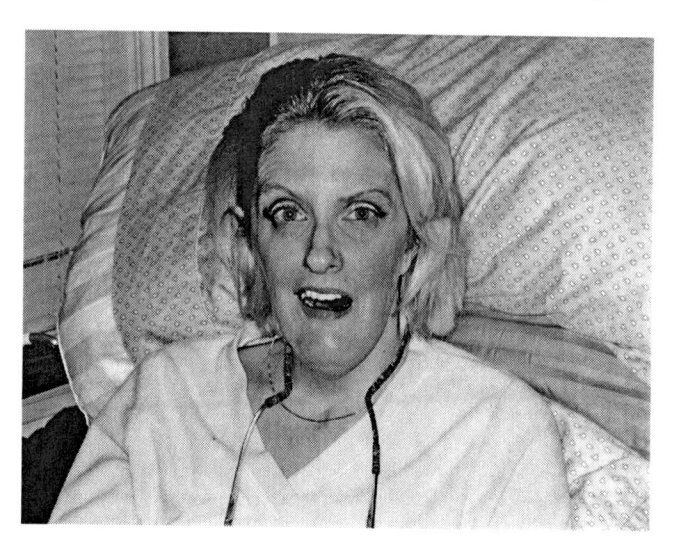

LOST SOME WEIGHT BUT GOOD TO BE ALIVE

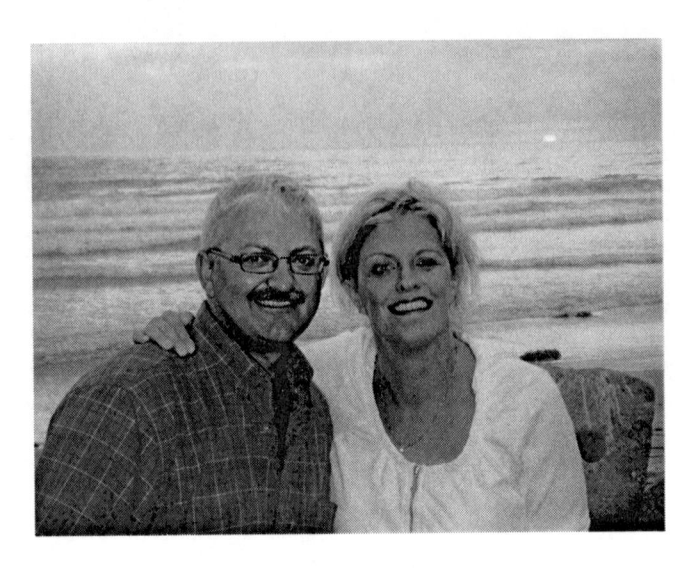

OUR LAST SAN DIEGO VACATION JUST PRIOR TO STROKE

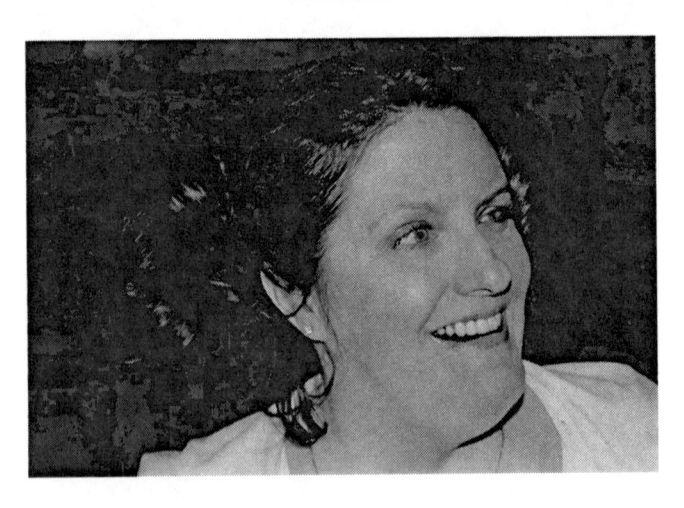

GETTING BACK TO NORMAL...ALL GOOD

Chapter Six

A Brighter Day

The next day, much to our surprise, Sandy's long awaited guests did show up! We were both shocked, but delighted. Oh how I wished that I had been told they would still be coming this very weekend. It would have saved so much heartache for my wife, and she was in such rough shape at this point. We never knew if there would even be a tomorrow.

When someone, anyone, is in the position that Sandy was in, it becomes difficult to deal with the passage of time. It is incredibly difficult to deal with the repetitious and slow moving day to day routine. It breaks you down.

In a very real sense, it was like living through the movie *Groundhog Day*. Routine, routine and more routine. When you cannot measure headway in a significant form of recovery, time passes ever so slowly.

Everyone handles sickness and grief in his or her own way. For some, the thought of spending time with a loved one in the hospital is perhaps just too difficult to bear. At least this is what we told ourselves. We had a couple of family members tell us they were just too busy. They had husbands, they had jobs, holidays to take, classes for the kids.

The problem for us would reluctantly be in part, having to redefine our definition of family. Over time, we truly discovered who in our lives really cared. There were those who sacrificed, who gave as much as they could. My daughter gave up her career, a relationship, and came from out of town every weekend no matter what the weather, to comfort us on a regular basis and to assist with the running of our home. She became our rock and we are so proud of her. It was especially difficult for us the day my children came over and gave us a financial love gift. Can you say proud?

※

More Angels

To all of those wonderful souls who brought chicken soup, meat pies, fresh bread, homemade desserts and physically held us when I, myself, could no longer stand; to those who organized events to help with our cash flow, cried with us, laughed with us, hurt with us and rejoiced with us, we thank you! The kindness we were shown, even by complete strangers, goes beyond comprehension and restored our faith. We promised ourselves if we ever made it through this mess, we would do our best to make a positive difference in this world.

These days, the wounds of emotional hurt have lessened; but the scars remain. Both of us must continue to work at restoring a few family relationship casualties. We have certainly made our fair share of mistakes along the way, and for this we truly say we're sorry. In order to move on, we all must forgive any wrongs whether real or perceived. We have to keep reminding ourselves daily that as difficult and as catastrophic as this has been, there are many others in this world who are suffering similar fates or are in much worse circumstances.

I recall one late evening in particular when I entered the elevator on the fourth floor and was heading down to the lobby. The elevator was almost filled to capacity; yet no one spoke. Perhaps many like me, were just feeling the stress of leaving a loved one and were exhausted; or perhaps pressed for anything positive to share, each of us were kind of hoping no one would speak. One floor down, the elevator doors opened and a young gentleman asked if he could squeeze in. Wheeling himself in all by himself, despite only having one leg, we pressed together to accommodate him.

"How y'all doin'?" he would ask us as he navigated the quickly closing doors. Breaking the silence, I asked him where he was heading and why the big hurry.

In an upbeat voice, he replied he was heading outside to get some fresh air. Adding that this might be his last trip outside for a while, he went on to explain that first thing in the morning they were going to take off his *other* leg. You could have heard a pin drop! And with that, he left us with a final word..."Have had great day!" Enough said.

Let me digress for a moment and take you back to one of the early days when one of the night nurses tried cleaning the inside of Sandy's mouth with a foam stick. Because Sandy was being tube fed, her mouth would naturally dry out. Sandy suddenly gagged and instinctively clamped down tightly. The only problem was that her tongue was in the way! I jumped from the chair and immediately began trying to pry her jaws apart; but it was extremely difficult. I, too, was panicking along with the nurse who at this point was shouting for me not to put my fingers into Sandy's mouth for fear of having them bitten off. With blood pouring from both sides of her mouth and her tongue sticking out, I had visions of Sandy biting off the tip of her tongue.

I still have all of my fingers. Sandy still has her tongue; which is a good thing because biting it off would have been a real added problem with her speech. I thought to myself, what else could possibly go wrong?

At this point I was beginning to wonder just how much more Sandy could take. We fought constantly with her lungs filling up with fluid. Again, no matter how far Sandy would come as far as moving her limbs went, there was always a tight rope we seemed to be walking. Often I would think we were on the verge of a major breakthrough, only to be let down with news that Sandy was back in the ICU.

There would be many challenging and hair-raising moments to follow in the coming days, weeks and months. But through it all, Sandy had one constant focus: "I do not have time for the *what if's*", she would often communicate to me, adding "let's make tomorrow today".

It was during these difficult days that our cousins held a special fundraising gala for us. There was a tremendous turnout in Saint Albert, and the proceeds went a long way towards the anticipated completion of the renovations needed for Sandy's return home. We will never forget the kindness and generosity of all who attended. We did make a brief visit to the hall, but could not stay long because we were overcome with emotion.

The following is so true. If on your deathbed, you were to be asked what was important in life, it would no doubt be the support and past memories of family and friends who stood by you during the tough times. It would be relationships and moments shared together through good times and bad. You would not be wondering whether or not the house work was done, or how much money you had in the bank.

I remember Christmas approaching and sitting in the hospital. For us it was just another day in the year; but, of course, it also had special meaning. Now the focus was on things that really mattered--not what was under the tree but who was around it.

≈≈

The Best Gifts of All

Hospitals are different at Christmas time, because the wards all but clear out except for the very sick. At this point Sandy was showing signs of improvement. Her right arm could fully extend upwards and she could, for the first time, touch the top of her head. She was also gaining strength and use of the fingers on her right hand. I remember thinking that perhaps I should not place any heavy objects in her tiny hand because she always had pretty good aim.

Sandy's left thumb and index finger were also beginning to show signs of life; and at times she even had enough strength to gently move her left arm forward!

December went by very quickly, and Sandy had many visitors from out of town. I believe it was the first week in January when we ventured out into the large and beautiful atrium area located directly beside Sandy's ward. It was good for Sandy to be sitting, as opposed to lying in her bed; and since she had not fainted in quite some time, off we went. I informed the nursing station where we would be and for how long. We would just take a short stroll.

It was at this point, that Sandy could even slightly move her left foot, shrug her shoulders and point. She used to take her right hand and grab her left wrist, stretching her forearm forward. This brought tremendous relief and gave her a feeling she could to some extent begin looking after her own needs. She could even scratch her itchy scalp.

There we were, proud as punch, as I wheeled Sandy into the beautiful sunlit atrium which was still festively decorated. There were groups of nurses and doctors milling about. The plants were thriving from the vast glass ceiling. The sun was shining and with everyone in the party mood, we moved on to find our own little neck of the woods.

We found our spot and parked along the rail which overlooked the area below us. We no sooner got the IV pole situated when Sandy began to topple over in her wheelchair. It's okay....just a balancing thing. Sandy, over time, would use her head to compensate for this problem. She would literally tilt from left or right depending on which way she was leaning.

No sooner had we arrived and got settled, when I noticed Sandy staring at a rather large group of doctors and nurses who were congregating in one of the open seating areas just to our immediate right. They were all smiling from ear to ear when they saw Sandy; and many were waving and giving her the thumbs up. How did my Sandy respond? She gave them the finger! I nearly melted into the carpet. Unfortunately Sandy had not yet mastered the fine art of hand/finger control. We quickly left the area.

We were hopeful that the many forms we were requested to complete for long term care down the road would not be required. Our focus at this point was to get Sandy to the much acclaimed Glenrose Rehabilitation Hospital as soon as possible. It would be another two months before this would happen; but it was all Sandy could think about. She was determined to get rid of her second trachea. A situation that would have to be resolved prior to moving forward on any rehabilitation centre.

In the meantime, I continued to prepare our home with a special bed, and converted our dining room into one of the sweetest hospital rooms you could ever imagine. Our buffet became the medical centre and hub for our caregivers. Curtains were installed for Sandy's privacy. We were able to acquire IV Poles and tables from the Red Cross. The roll in shower would have to wait for a few months; but we intended to tackle this next project during the Glenrose stay.

Our main goal was to put Sandy in a position where she could come home on some of the weekends during the expected rehab process. We had heard that they let some people "escape" providing they went back. In time, we would make this work; and the Glenrose would assist us by providing us with all of the necessary advice on getting our home up to code.

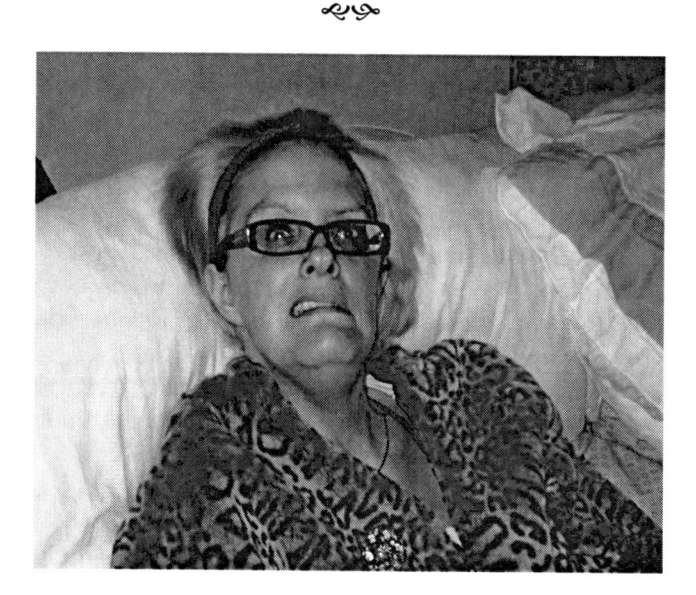

ALWAYS THE FASHION QUEEN

Sandy's Thoughts

Going over this chapter reminded me once again just how fortunate we are to have such supportive extended family and friends in our lives. It gave me comfort to know that David was being fed; that he too had people around him holding him up. I had heard too many horror stories of caregivers burning out and knew that we were in a Marathon, not a sprint. I drew strength from simply hearing of the many acts of random kindness. At times it overwhelmed me and those near us thought I was depressed. There would be many moments when I would cry out of appreciation and respect for our circle of support.

Courtesy of me, Dave was introduced to the ICU ward several times. I remember Dave talking to me about how scared he was the first time. He apparently witnessed them covering up someone across from my room who didn't make it. Then someone inadvertently left a curtain open and when he looked up from comforting me on the stretcher, he witnessed the aftermath of someone who had lost both of his legs and family members were all gathered around.

My husband always said that he wasn't sure if he could go through what I have been through. He said that he would like to think he could have switched places with me; but I am glad that it was I, and not he, who suffered the effects of a stroke. He is a big baby and his complaining would have driven everyone completely insane. The only positive thing might have been an early discharge from the hospital.

∽∾

Chapter Seven

The Escape

Sandra's stay in the University Hospital lasted six months. After two failed attempts to remove her trachea tube, she was to be third time lucky. No longer confined, we had the green light to commence a more aggressive therapy program at the Glenrose Rehabilitation Hospital. Both Sandy and I were absolutely thrilled! There they would work on things such as balance, walking, standing, speaking, dressing, hand co-ordination and the ultimate goal...washroom independence.

It was official. In the morning, Sandy would be heading to the Glenrose Rehabilitation Hospital via inter ambulance transfer. Dr. Hamadeh, Sandy's primary doctor from day one, made a special trip to the ward tonight just to say goodbye to Sandy one last time.

It was strange to see him in street apparel, baseball cap and all. He was always impeccably groomed and a sharp dresser; Professional with a capital P. The sight of him dressed so casually seemed very fitting as it was time to move on and enjoy living. Hope for the future was all around us.

Sandy told me that she will miss his daily visits where for so long he would enter the room, walk over to Sandy's side and ask her to say...."Ah." Then, like a coach, he would bend down, look into her eyes and say, "now louder Sandy....can you say 'ah' louder?" For the longest time nothing much came out; but then little by little, Sandy got the hang of it. That was a major step!

I recall one day when Sandy asked me why Dr. Hamadeh always talked so loudly to her? "Does he think I am deaf as well?" I laughed my head off because this was something that he did…every time!

When we finally told Dr. Hamadeh what Sandy had said, he took it in stride, and we caught a little chuckle. "Okay", he said, "I'll try to remember that, Sandy."

I'm sure the good doctor was happy to see me go as well because I used to track him down in the halls before he made good his escape from his long days in the hospital. Many times, just seeing this doctor one last time before the end of the day would be enough to help Sandy settle down for the evening. I must say, he sure had a way with Sandy!

Sandy was still battling with some breathing issues but they assured us that a suction airline would be made available to her when she arrived at her awaiting private room. There they would have the skilled and talented folks who would assist Sandy by developing and designing fancy leg and hand braces--tools that would make her life "easier". There would be an overhead lift in her room to make it easier for the necessary transfers from her bed to her wheelchair. Initially we were told that this would be a semi-private room. One thing for sure, it was going to be boot camp.

I remember feeling very emotional that last night. Everyone who knows us, knows how emotional both Sandy and I can get, and this was such a huge day. Some of the nurses escaped my hugs that night but there was not a dry eye on the ward when I made the final trip downstairs to the van with the last of Sandy's room contents.

Over the past six months, Sandy's room had become somewhat of a shrine; overloaded with cards, stuffed animals and gifts of all sorts. It seemed odd having to leave Sandy behind; but by the time everything was crammed inside, there was really only enough room left for me in the van. There was protocol that had to be followed and the hospital staff assured me that they would get her safely to the Glenrose and that the journey by ambulance was necessary.

I arrived back home and plunked myself down into my desk chair. Staring at my computer I was afraid to even open it; for fear of the hundreds of emails that would be awaiting my attention. Clients would be wondering if I would be returning to work. Friends and family eagerly awaiting the next update on Sandy's progress and there would be emails from our website inquiring how things were progressing. Last, but not least, was the pressure I put on myself to stay on top of everything.

I remember getting up from my chair and deciding to unload the van and bring the contents into our home office. Sitting back down, I decided to write a short email to everyone sharing the good news that Sandy will be transferred to the Glenrose. As I began to type, I looked down at a box containing many of the cards Sandy had received. I looked at a large pile of string, now tangled in a huge ball that once held these notes and precious get well cards. It seemed like a fitting analogy to our life. It was all there….we just had to unravel it.

※

Life at the Glenrose Hospital

As time would progress, Sandy would eventually wear everything out. When asked to do anything, Sandy would always push further and harder. She would press herself to the limits of exhaustion. Although Sandy would come all too soon to realize and accept that she had also lost peripheral vision and she would never drive again, this would not stop her from achieving her goals. She would walk again. She would swallow again. She would speak again. This was our ticket, her chance, her moment. We were off to the highly respected Glenrose Rehabilitation Hospital.

We were introduced to a whole new staff and quickly evolved into higher expectations, and a little more independence. This would be our new home for the next five and a half months. Much to our delight, the nurses, doctors and the therapists all surpassed our expectations. We are truly blessed to have a facility such as this. Without these dedicated souls many would suffer agonizing defeat and have no alternative but to be institutionalized.

It really was a team effort and both hospitals extended great love and guidance, and just the right amount of push! After the Glenrose, Sandy would receive additional ongoing therapy at the CRIS clinic. Many of these professionals would touch our lives in ways we never imagined.

Looking back, much of our routine, or should I say my routine, remained the same in that I would go to the hospital early in the morning and leave late at night. I began working mornings for a while, but the late nights caught up with me and eventually the business of over thirty years would come to an end; as would our finances. We certainly had our problems juggling the money. In fact, on one occasion when Sandy was having her trachea replaced, and during the hysteria, her front tooth was accidentally pulled out in the process! More bills to come I would think. Next!

As if this was not bad enough, just days later, I lost my front tooth as well. I will never forget the moment when I walked into Sandra's room and gave her the big grin. She howled with laughter. I thought to myself, what on earth are the odds of this happening to us at the same time? What a sight for sore eyes we were!

Actually it did have one small benefit. When people would stare at Sandy while I rolled her down the hallways, I would whisper to Sandy to smile and we would both put on our widest grins at the same time just as we passed their wide eyeballs. Generally this would do the trick and the staring would end. I was very happy when the hospital agreed to replace Sandra's front tooth at their expense. For your viewing pleasure, we have included a picture of our smiling mugs.

We would share many of these stories at the end of the day when, as mentioned before, Sandy's Aunt Nadia would appear with muffins and coffee in hand. Truly we worried about her when she did not come by, as we knew she always wanted to provide family comfort to Sandy. In fact Nadia's daughter Roberta, who, as luck would have it, is a nurse, also saw Sandy on a regular basis in the Glenrose Hospital. She would often stop by to comfort Sandy in those lonely early mornings just following her night shift in a nearby wing. Without question, there were angels all around Sandy!

≈≋≈

Trying to be Normal

It was to be our first trip into the general public since Sandy's injury. We headed to West Edmonton Mall via the DATS Handicap Bus Service. It would only be a few hours; but this was a huge day for Sandy. I took her to a salon to have her hair done. She was reluctant at first; but we did eventually get Sandy to look in the mirror. She seemed pleased with her new look. While at the mall, we picked out a few new outfits for Sandy. I should have checked the prices; but it was worth every dime to see Sandy smiling.

Once our excursion was finished, we headed back down to the prearranged pick up spot. While waiting for the DATS bus, I removed Sandy's leg braces, hung them on the back of her power wheelchair and rubbed her little feet. The braces caused her a great deal of pain and swelling; but prevented her feet from curling outwards, worse than they already were. Thank God this inversion and twisting of her feet would later be addressed!

We encountered just one unpleasant experience on the bus when a young girl panicked and started howling. Apparently she was alarmed thinking that she was going to be removed from the bus. It was in fact our stop. The caregiver or travel companion did little, no make that nothing, to comfort her. I made eye contact with the gal and assured her that this was not her stop and that all would be okay. It was hard to leave the bus after that.

Despite the crowds and the constant staring at us, all in all, it was still a good day. For the life of me, I really wonder at times what the heck is wrong with some people. There are always those that for whatever reason, feel they must stare. It's like the deer in the headlight look--frozen in time. That said, I would absolutely love it when Sandy would return the eye contact and twist her face up like a prune as I would wheel her past everyone. Priceless.

※

Sandy's Thoughts

This was truly the halfway point; but in many ways

entering the Glenrose Rehabilitation Center felt like the beginning. I was excited to learn how to regain some independence.

In particular, I was looking forward to having showers at the Glenrose Rehabilitation Hospital. I remember back to the early days when they would wheel me into the "Tub Room" at the U of A Hospital. The stretcher was some sort of hard cold plastic. I know it was just a few feet but my circulation was not the best and the ride along this short trip to the water was anything but pleasurable.

One day they asked David if he would like to help with my bathing routine and I was thinking that this might not be such a good idea as David gets distracted very easily. In fact it was actually a touching moment for us when Dave held my head up and watched the water line rise. He was so careful to not let a single drop of water enter my mouth although at one point I started to slip and he managed to completely soak himself from the waist down in the process. This would not have been such a big deal, but it was nighttime and snowing outside. I think he, too, was very glad for the progress I had made thus far, and the ability to now hold myself upright in a wheelchair. Being at the Glenrose would mean no more baths!

Being a self-proclaimed fashion queen, I must say I was relieved to finally be back into street clothes and regular apparel--one of the conditions of "living" at the Glenrose. Dave, however, in his infinite good taste, decided that for some ungodly reason I should have a wide array of hospital nurses' outfits. I believe he went shopping at a local drug store and picked out every color under the sun. The bolder the better! Well, at least they were easy outfits to put on; and all came with elastic waistbands. I even blended in with the staff. Oh yes...Dave had great style when it came to picking out my clothes but I never complained...until now.

I know David means well, but his idea of a successful shopping trip is measured by how quickly he can get back out. These days I take my caregivers along whenever possible. It's just better for our relationship.

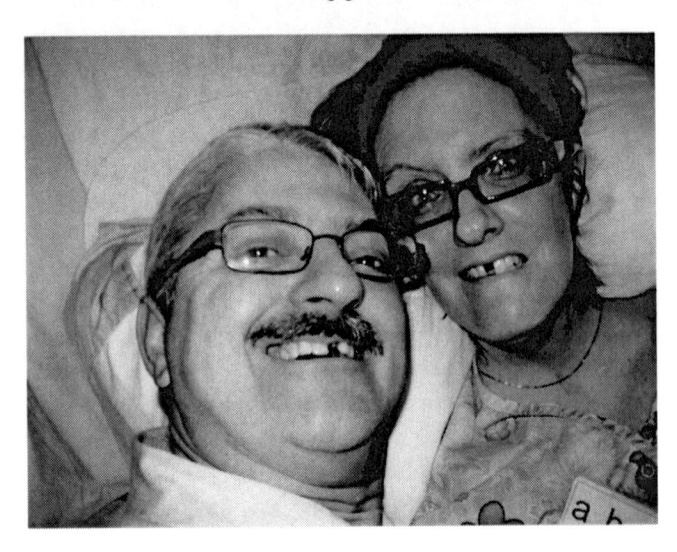

❦

SAY CHEESE

Chapter Eight

☙❧

Rehab

March 17, 2008 It was an exciting day. A day we were beginning to wonder would ever happen. It will be different now, we thought, and we were right. Sandy would actually be dressed every day and start to resemble the living. Gone were the days of Sandy's passing out when she would be lifted upright. Still such a long way to go, but at least now that light at the end of the tunnel was no longer a freight train staring us down.

Therapy sessions took up her entire day and when she wasn't working out, she would practise in bed. Sandy was a relentless student. She became an inspiration to all around her with her positive attitude and gentle persistence. Although there was still talk of Sandy being institutionalized down the road, we both knew she was coming home. I made Sandy a commitment and my not having our home renovations completed was never going to be an option. Of course it was Sandy who had the real job!

They even remembered to have Sandy put in a room which had a suction device. Apparently not too many rooms had one. The staff was on her as soon as she arrived discussing what would soon best be described as boot camp. We had no idea that it would be five and a half months before Sandy would be released from rehab. This would not be a quick process; such a long road ahead. Sandy was glad to be in the Glenrose despite being labelled a long-term resident; besides, we got a few good breaks on the TV rental.

The first night in the hospital felt strange but exhilarating. Sandy asked me to hold her. I held her close to my body, as tightly as I could without hurting her. Hugging was something we did all the time; but tonight was different. I sat her up, balanced her little body and we embraced for a long time.

Then Sandy asked for her letter board and she spelled out the following; "David, I'm so glad to be married to you." I choked back the tears and replied that I was the lucky one. I would marry Sandy a thousand times over. She had grown so much, in so many ways. She had shown such tremendous inner strength. She would still struggle with many health concerns and emotional swings in the days ahead; but who, I would often wonder, wouldn't, under these circumstances.

Communicating would prove to be one of Sandy's biggest challenges. Sometimes she would get frustrated when people did not understand what she was trying to say, and she would roll up her eyes and put the finger gun to her head, pulling the trigger and collapsing. We got the message loud and clear.

∽⚭∽

Weekend Pass

The house renovations would be extensive but necessary to help Sandy once she did get back home. We hired a full time contractor to carry out things like converting our storage room into a roll-in shower, removing carpet, installing hardwood, putting up privacy curtains in the dining room which would be her temporary bedroom, a ceiling lift, wheelchair accessible ramps and an elevator. Every window was coated with a thin film to filter out the bright sunshine that hurt her eyes.

At the same time, we did not want our home to look like a hospital. I think we achieved the desired look; because I'll never forget the day Sandy came home and the wonderful expression on her face. Sure these were just day visits at first, but institutional living would never be an option.

Speaking of weekend home visits, they did not happen until about the fourth month into her Glenrose stay. There were difficult emotional challenges, particularly when Sandy had to head back to the hospital. We came to dread Sunday nights; and as time would go on we would take her back to the prison, I mean hospital, later and later. Thankfully, the evening staff put up with our shenanigans. We never wanted the nurses to think we did not appreciate what they were doing for us. It's just that there's no place like home.

∞

A Simple Drive

Home visits always seemed to have the unexpected happen. We had so much to learn; so many new ways of having to adapt and do things; things that were once so easy to do--for instance, going for a drive together.

Sometimes, even returning to the Glenrose after a home visit proved to have its challenges. One night while waiting for the cab to arrive, we wondered if it *was* ever going to arrive. Just when we were about to give up hope, the cab appeared. There was just one problem. It was a regular cab and not equipped to transport the disabled.

I went out and talked to the cabdriver, explaining the situation, and asked how much longer we would have to wait. He's just stared at me with a blank look, muttering "I work for idiots" and drove away.

I quickly called the dispatcher back and explained that this was all previously arranged. I explained the urgency of Sandy needing to get back to the hospital for her night medications, thinking they might understand the urgency of meeting the hospital's directives and hoping it would make a difference! My words were falling on deaf ears. The dispatchers replied, "We're a cab company. What do you expect?" A number of retorts raced through my mind; but I bit my tongue and was glad in the end that I didn't sound off too much because a cab did show up that was able to meet our needs.

Perhaps my stressing to them that Sandra needed her scheduled evening medications played a part. Whatever the reason, we were just glad a replacement cab showed up. Just when I was thinking everything was 'a go', the driver quickly jumped out from the van and headed for the narrow space along our sloped driveway. He was facing the garage door and was completely motionless. Not only was he facing the garage door, but he was squeezed between a parked car and our retaining wall. We were concerned and watching the time but he left his hat on the roof of the car so we figured there was a pretty good chance he would return. Surely if he needed to use the washroom he would have asked. There was no need to use our outside drain I told Sandy in disgust. Just then, Terry, our neighbor and friend, came over to our window and informed us that the driver was *praying*. He must have been able to read the bewilderment on our faces and figured he should tell us what was going on. We were relieved.

This was to be a very "professional driver" as he would remind us every few miles. We had a safe trip home; but I could have walked faster. At one section of freeway, we were passed by a cyclist. At one red light we were almost swallowed by a semi. I think this driver figured when the light turned green, this meant wait another five minutes and say another prayer. I did ask him about the speed he was travelling and he quickly informed me that he was a "professional" and the posted traffic signs and signals did not apply to him. We hope and pray he is still alive.

There was a weekend when Sandra was at home and had been struggling with her secretions, and just in general, having a tough time. I remember it was about 4:00 p.m. and Sandra suggested that we should get out of the house for a bit. It sounded like a good idea; after all, our new van had finally arrived, complete with automatic ramp.

I mentioned to Sandy that that she looked a little swollen and suggested that it might be better if we waited for a while before venturing out. Sandy would have no part of this; stressing to me that all was well and there was no need to wait.

Looking back, I think we should have waited. I attempted to transfer Sandy into her wheelchair. In the process, I rolled her wheelchair over my foot and managed to completely wind our new soft white blanket around the wheel. By the looks of it, someone must have thought it was necessary to over grease the wheels as there were globs of grease hanging down everywhere. I turned my attention to Sandy, determined to get her off the bed and into the chair. Time was ticking by quickly.

Thinking nothing else could possibly go wrong, I once more attempted to lift Sandy off the bed and into the wheelchair. This time I managed to snag Sandy's feeding tube which was attached to her tummy, and it came flying out, spurting all the contents from Sandy's last lunch. We took approximately the next forty minutes to both get cleaned up and changed. Had I been able to find the clip, which had magically vaporized, to hold the tube shut, the transfer would have gone a whole lot more smoothly.

Backing up, I somehow managed to wheel the chair over Sandy's left foot. As though on cue, Sandy lifted her little fist into the air, gave it a shake, expressing to me just how great this felt. Sandy just grinned and chuckled at my clumsiness. She is so forgiving and takes everything in stride; and I'm sure at this point, like me, she just wanted to get out of the house.

I, too, was anxious to get into the air conditioned van. The sweat was profusely streaming down my face and my back; and as a rule, I don't sweat much. I was completely exhausted. We were finally ready to leave and load Sandy onto our elevator. Naturally, the elevator did not move. We couldn't believe this was happening. Over and over again, we played with the levers. Much like lifting the engine hood of a car, we expected it to repair itself; and amazingly it suddenly worked! We were free at last!

I followed Sandy down using the stairs; and just before exiting I turned on the alarm. At least that was the idea. Surprise! It didn't work, either. I locked the door and left in disgust.

We were in our garage and I could sense Sandy looking at me. She was very quiet. Our shiny new black van was to be our freedom, our escape from this madness. Like a magician, I pulled the key fob from my pocket and aimed it like a wand towards this awesome looking marvel.

Having just arrived from the dealer, our new wheels looked great. The skilled technicians who did the conversion down south really knew their stuff. The long wait for this magnificent piece of mechanical beauty would all be worth it.

At the press of a button, the engine rumbled and the doors began to open like something out of *Star Trek*. Following the opening of the side door, the gray coated steel ramp extended towards Sandy like a welcome mat. We were seemingly on a roll, and a drive looked eminent.

I walked around the back of the wheelchair, grabbed the handles and prepared to take one last dash up the ramp and into the van. I suddenly put on the brakes! For some ungodly reason, as if Murphy had gone wild, the ramp ceased to come out, and recoiled into the van. I pressed the button again, and as if to taunt us, it came back--all but four inches. These few inches may not seem like a big deal but when the wheelchair's and patient's weights are combined, there is no way you're getting on that ramp if it has not lowered properly. While this was all happening, I was thinking about the $72,000 debt with which we had been blessed. Enough time had been wasted, so I decided to crawl into the van and start cranking by hand to get the ramp down and Sandy into the vehicle. While cranking the ramp back into the van, my knees throbbing in pain, I wondered just how wise an investment this was. I also wondered how in the world someone in a wheelchair would do what I had just done.

By this time, it was time to head back to the Glenrose and get Sandy settled for the night. Needless to say our drive was not very long. Arriving at our destination, and parking the van in their underground parkade, almost seemed a relief. I remember walking around the van in disgust and thinking what a disaster our day had been.

Opening the door to Sandy, I was soon to discover our night was not over. Somehow the mechanical geniuses who designed the van messed up with the seat belts; of course it was just Sandy's side. Instead of loosening, it grew increasingly tighter. I tried to slide the seat back while tilting Sandy's wheelchair. This proved to be an effective ligature and did nothing to help free her. The shoulder restraint was now tight against her chest and sliding up her neck which only made things worse.

Once more I was beginning to sweat, and not really sure what to do. I screamed for a nurse who was walking by. Thankfully she heard our cries for help, ran back into the hospital and brought back one of the largest pair of shears I had ever seen. I had no idea at the time that this seat belt would have to be replaced at a cost of $750.00 plus labor. We eventually took a financial loss on the mini-van and sold it. We both prayed that the new owners would have better luck with it than we had.

The Home Escapes

Not all weekends were a disaster. Over time, we would look at these as just minor bumps in the road. As a rule, we would just laugh and try to make the best of any situation. I recall one such weekend when we had no sooner gotten into the house and Sandy asked to sit on our newly upholstered loveseat. Sitting in a normal chair since we were at home, just seemed appropriate.

Sitting there together on the loveseat brought back many good memories. I rubbed her feet and for just a brief moment it seemed like old times. Then I glanced over and looked at her wheelchair in front of our fireplace. It didn't matter that it shared the room; we were enjoying the moment and at least for now, things felt normal.

As previously mentioned, we had converted our dining room into a temporary bedroom. This avoided any stairs and provided easy access no matter what time of day. Our dear friends, Derek and Kathy, along with Shirley and Roy, had made custom curtains for us which ran on a ceiling track. If you add a hydraulic bed, IV pole, power ceiling lift and medical supplies, you have the perfect hospital away from the hospital room.

I no sooner had Sandy comfortable in her bed when she told me that what she'd really like to do was to see the renovated washrooms and the upstairs! I figured what the heck? I'm Sampson, I can do it. I picked her up and hoisted her as high as possible over my back. I needed to get a good grip on Sandy without hurting her as there were a total of sixteen steps in front of me. I thought to myself that the hospital staff would die if they saw this; but it would be our little secret. After all, I knew Sandy would be thrilled to see the renovated upstairs bathrooms.

Okay, we were ready to go. Holding Sandy firmly, I gave one last upwards thrust, positioning her securely in my arms. With this last thrust, her glasses went flying. Realizing that this was not a good thing and that she was now as blind as a bat I was quick to realize that even if I were now able to get her upstairs, she wouldn't be able to see anything anyway. Obviously I needed to grab her glasses; and in a panic at the moment, I didn't really know quite what to do. There we were frozen in time. After much contemplation, I gently lowered her and with one arm explored for her fallen glasses. At this point, Sandy was dangling high over my shoulder. She was laughing hysterically, her eyes wet with tears. I was actually concerned about the neighbors who must surely be wondering what was going on in the Nette household.

With both of us laughing the energy I once thought I had to achieve this task, was quickly disappearing. I felt every muscle in my body. Needless to say, we had to abandon this idea, and leave looking at the upstairs washrooms until my back healed.

It was also during this time that we had a number of meetings with specialists regarding Sandy's ankles. Her feet continued to curl down and point towards the floor. They had also twisted over time and were almost fully inverted. We were faced with the realization that even if Sandy could walk, her feet would be useless; but more on this later.

∼∽

Workouts

Therapists must possess great patience and have thick skin. Their skills often honed over time. In the way, they are counsellors as well; probably as a result of dealing with such serious injuries and many stroke victims. They're the best!

The whole atmosphere of being in a rehab center is so much better than a regular hospital setting. Both serve their purpose; but for many, rehab is a sign of hope. It's difficult to have faith when just taking a breath of air is a challenge. Sandy went over a year without taking anything by mouth, not even the smallest teaspoon of water. Just try and imagine that for a second. Can you say gross?

Of all the things lost, privacy would remain high on Sandy's list. When one depends on twenty-four hour care, dignity must be put aside. To this day, this loss of control over her world continues to cause her sadness. It is one of the most difficult aspects of Sandy's stroke.

Over time with every small victory, no matter how minor, everyone would rejoice enthusiastically. All the therapists coordinated their efforts like a professional sports team, with one unified goal. They all work in perfect harmony trying to achieve the very best results and gaining as much independence as was possible for every patient.

◈

Sandy's Thoughts

Hmm...looking back I am wondering how David managed to stay positive about these home visits. It seemed as if something off the wall was almost a certainly going to happen. These moments, although somewhat taxing at the time, did provide us with interesting reflection.

I truly believe that it's important to maintain at least some sense of humour during difficult times. Laughter for me provided a pressure relief valve; and David did not "seem" to mind being the focus of much of my hysterical laughter.

I knew when I was dating David and we took a whale watching tour, that he was the man for me. The Zodiac had two huge outboard motors hanging off the back end (stern, port, helm, rear, whatever you call it) and the boat flew along the waves like a speeding bullet. I could barely keep my eyes open when the captain hit full throttle. We had the front row seat all to ourselves with the rest of the people all crowded in behind us like sardines. I will never forget how exciting and romantic this was for me...that was until Dave asked me what I thought would happen if he spit his large wad of gum out. Yes...I knew right then and there that this was the man for me.

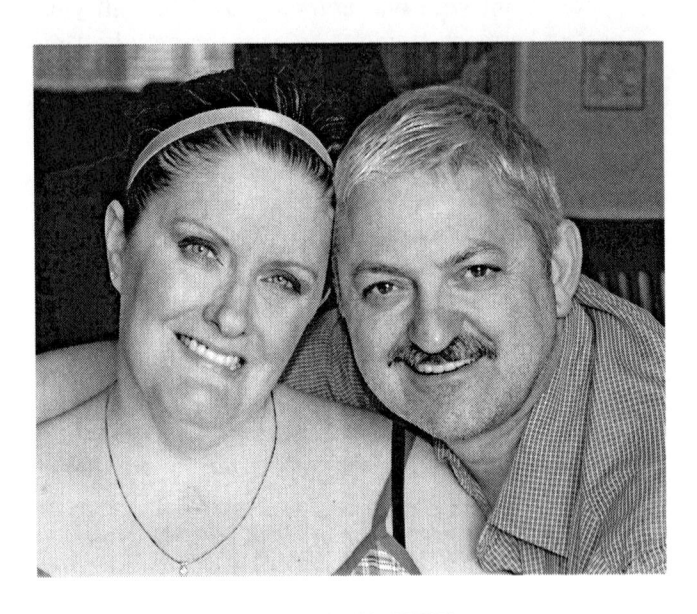

I LOVE SANDY'S EYES!

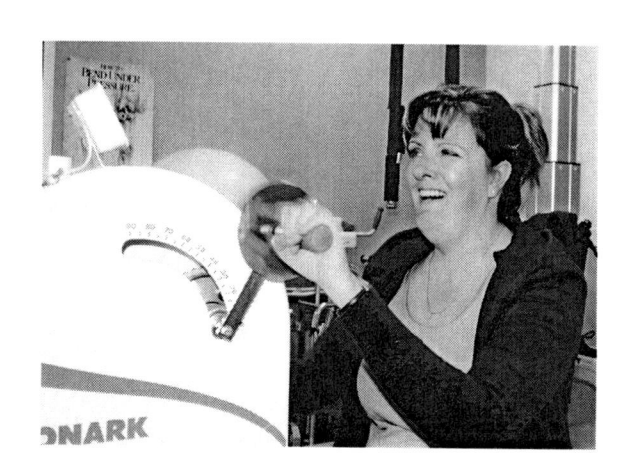

I ACTUALLY LIKE THIS THING

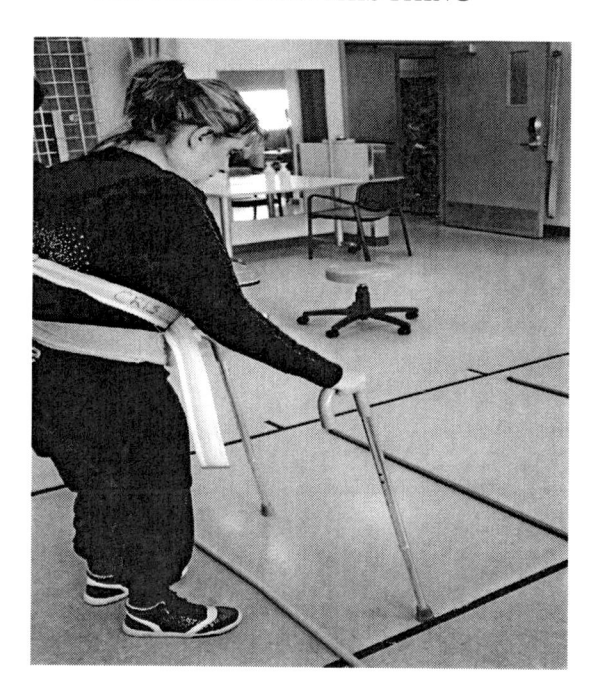

BABY STEPS

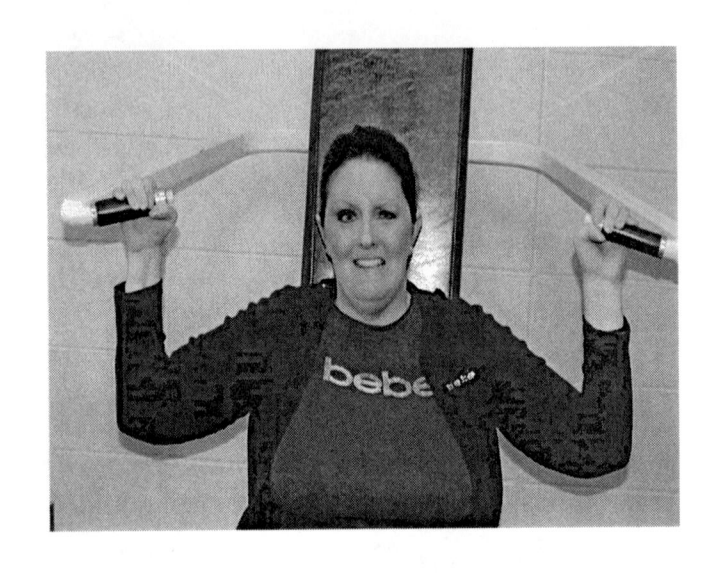

YOU GO GIRL

Chapter Nine

※

Million Dollar Baby

Although I enjoyed getting Sandy back home at any opportunity, the weekends could be a little tough; so there were nights when I was more tired than usual. One particular weekend we had a small miracle, no make that a BIG miracle!

Sandy was having a little bit of trouble with some sour reflux. Her energy level was very low and the head nurse requested we purchase a blood pressure tester and monitor her levels while she was away from the hospital. We had no problem doing this as we certainly didn't want to take any chances. Sandy had been through enough already.

Sandy had her new "leopard" leg braces fitted and they looked terrific. They gave her support to stand and prevented her ankles from turning outwards. Enabling Sandy to stand upright was quite a treat. It had been so long since we had stared at each other eyeball to eyeball.

It was this weekend that we tried to experiment a little with her ability to swallow. Sandy wanted to try to swallow again. I was very nervous but agreed to try something. With my daughter, Linda, by my side we went to the kitchen, took a small can of peaches and fired up the blender. I'm sure Sandy was wondering what exactly was going on, as it had been such a long time since anything had been attempted in this manner. I had suction equipment standing by just in case something went down the wrong pipe. Strangely, Sandy did not appear to have any issues; except things did get a little messy. I had never been so happy to do laundry.

The trick to this feat was to use one of Sandy's mouth cleansing sponges. Picture a small swab with a foam end on it. We would soak up the excess using the sponge. In total, it took about forty-five minutes for Sandy to consume two ounces. We all sat there stunned. Although I knew the hospital would give us heck, we just had to try to do it again.

In the months that followed, Sandy would be retrained to swallow. It took a very long time; but eventually Sandy would get to the point where she could eat once again and no longer need the stomach tube. Water was perhaps the most difficult thing for Sandy to swallow because it is so thin.

Just as important as the act of eating and being able to enjoy a good meal, was the socializing aspect that accompanied these times. We loved to entertain as a couple and spent much of our time in the kitchen. I would do the cooking and Sandy would add her flare by co-ordinating every single detail right down to the music. It would be a matter of time, but we would get back there.

To date, over two million dollars have been spent courtesy of the government, rebuilding Sandy. The numerous surgeries, long term hospital stays, medications, therapy, transportation, caregivers, speech therapists, psychologists, neurosurgeons, specialists, maxillofacial surgeons, orthopedic surgeons, etc., all continue to add up to one enormous cost.

Fun At The Dentist

It was June 19th 2008. Sandy just had a great day with her favorite dentist, Dr. Elisabeth Specht. This terrific dentist even shared her birthday cake with Sandy. After so many sessions of trying to prepare Sandy for her front tooth replacement they had grown very close.

I had no idea how complicated this front bridge work was going to be. A major part of the problem was that following the stroke, Sandy had limited mobility in her jaw. While Sandy never had a great opening, things were much worse since her stroke. The difficulty that this presented for the dentist was substantial, and it was not easy for Sandy, either. Four trips later and Sandy had spent a total of fifteen hours visiting the dentist. They guesstimated two more, hopefully short visits, and she'd be finished. She had undergone over thirty hours of completed dental preparation.

What a gruelling task. Frankly, I did not know how this dentist was doing it! We would both be glad when Sandy was finished with the dental procedures and could smile once more.

We arrived home and it was just another typical day. Sandy was exhausted and I needed to get her to bed. The air was sticky and the room was hot. I quickly made an adjustment to the power bed only to hear the snapping off of the extension cord's ground post. Time to slow down, I thought to myself.

The bed was too close to the wall; and in the process of making further adjustments, I tripped over the footrest supports of the wheelchair. I stumbled to the supply cabinet to collect the tools of the trade to get Sandy ready for some much needed rest.

Out of the corner of my eye, I noticed Sandy chuckling to herself. She took some sort of sick satisfaction in watching me fumble my way around. At least she was laughing, and I carried on.

For some reason, the room felt even hotter now; but perhaps it was just me. I took the opportunity to cover Sandy with baby powder. Then like an Einstein, I hit the power switch on the fan in one last attempt to cool things down. Big mistake! Once the fog lifted and I brushed myself off I looked at Sandy. It looked as though she had on a face mask. She was not amused.

My only excuse for why so many things went a little crazy that day might have been connected, or so I thought, when I walked headfirst into the exterior's top door frame of the van. I ran up that ramp like I owned the place; only to come to an abrupt stop as my forehead slammed against the metal opening. The stars were shining brightly.

Perhaps I had suffered a brain concussion. Obviously I needed to slow down. Obviously I had far too many things on my mind; including a nice sized goose egg. It seemed as if never a day went by without something happening. It was nonstop.

Sandy was going to be introduced to some new routines next week, to try to assist with the stomach and drinking issues. She would also be going to the Royal Alexandra Hospital to try the swallowing test again. The crunch was on to fit in as much as possible over the next six weeks. Sandy always looked forward to 4:00 p.m. when her routine would end and she would get a chance to go outside with me for a while. It was during this time that we were anxiously awaiting the green light to come home. We knew it would be a few months yet; but we didn't want to rush Sandy's therapy because we were seeing such great results.

I was constantly looking into the twenty-four hour home care that was available. I had made it my business to oversee every aspect of Sandy's health and well-being from day one.

I would be hiring family as well as few non family members to fill these caregivers' spots; therefore, I had made it my priority to provide as much background and input as possible in order for the staff we hired to do their job effectively. There were no manuals that we could simply hand out on managing Sandy's ever-changing day to day needs. Even the staff's personalities had to jell as this would ultimately be a tight group, often working side by side.

The house was almost complete, right down to the medical alert button. We even installed a portable air cleaner for the home in order to assist Sandy with her breathing. Now all I needed was Sandy.

❧

The Nine Month Mark

Sandy and I have always been what I would consider good communicators. She talked, I listened. Sandy heard me writing this and burst out laughing. The truth is that I talk a lot--sometimes too much. It was at the nine month mark, at the Glenrose that on many occasions I found myself completely hoarse. My throat was as dry as sandpaper from talking. There were still so many questions I had for Sandy and so much she wanted to tell me.

Although I rented a TV for her hospital room, Sandy rarely watched it. She preferred "talking". The hospital communication department had provided Sandy with a fancy voice board which was able to be attached to her wheelchair and was removable when needed elsewhere. It provided Sandy with a sexy female voice and all she had to do was press the appropriate letter. When the board worked, we would go on a frenzied spelling marathon. Past, present and future topics were all open game for this chicky poo. By the way, for some strange reason, the TV remote kept disappearing. Strange…very strange.

During this rehabilitation period, we still had a few other health concerns. For one thing, Sandy kept fainting--and it wasn't from my good looks. We were worried because it was in this month that she had, as far as we knew, fainted three times. Any thoughts of Sandy driving her car ever again were put to rest. Just as well, because I hated being the passenger, even though Sandy was a confident and fully capable driver no matter what the road conditions. Even if we could correct the fainting; the day was coming when Sandy would have to admit that this stroke had also permanently affected her peripheral vision.

This, however, didn't stop Sandy from driving altogether. This was the month that Sandy received a power wheelchair. This loaner was a hot rod! No one was safe once Sandy got into the seat. The hallway cleared; people ducked for cover and linen racks toppled over as Sandy grabbed the throttle stick and selected the "Rabbit". The "Rabbit", for those uninitiated, is the fastest speed possible on this mid-engine baby.

With time, Sandy got the hang of the chair and loved the independence it gave her. This chair also had a tilt action so that she could relieve pressure points on her body. Of course, any time a person is sitting upright as opposed to lying in bed, means a better future. Even one's lungs function better.

With time, they would teach Sandy how to drive more slowly; and to control her passion for speed. They would lay out obstacle pylons both inside the hospital and outside in the parking lot. For the first while, it would best be described as bumper cars. In time, Sandy would go on to have her very own chair. Unfortunately, it was even faster.

As for Sandy's progress, they continued to work on her leg braces trying to come up with a better design.

The staff in the Orthopedic Department was simply amazing! They even designed a small brace for Sandy's left hand which helped with the inward curling of the fingers. They always treated all of their patients with the utmost respect. This is one hospital that has seen its share of trauma survivors. Attitude is everything with these highly trained hospital staff members.

The Ups and the Downs

Sandy was transferred through the long underground hospital passageways at the ninth month mark and underwent another swallowing test. The news was not good; and the x-rays revealed that Sandy failed the test. This depressing news was absolutely devastating; but not completely unexpected. As Sandy was wheeled into the room where I was waiting, I could tell that the news was not good. Her contorted facial expression and the tears said it all.

"We will try this again, Sandy; and there will come a day when you will eat and drink again; a time when we will be able to say goodbye to the stomach feeding tube." Sandy calmed down without the use of any drugs; and we just held each other for a long, long time. This would just be another setback but not the final word.

We were not sure when they would attempt the swallowing tests again; but we knew that it would not be for a while. Sandy was also experiencing serious reflux issues, which added to her secretion issues. The last thing we wanted was to have her readmitted to the University of Alberta Hospital.

It was times like this, whether in the hospital or at home, when we would find ourselves alone with reality hitting us in the face. There would be many obstacles to overcome; but Sandy was as determined as ever to push her body back to health. Her stamina and stubborn determination would eventually pay off; but the challenges seemed out of our control. That night we requested oxygen; because her vitals had dropped to a dangerously low level. Once again, Sandy walked the edge.

Amazingly Sandy woke up the next day and it was as though she had regained a second wind. Perhaps it was the thought of coming home for the weekend. I don't know what caused the extreme turnaround; but when Sandy was put in the passenger side of the new van and the sun roof opened, it was as though she were in heaven. Just like in past times, we drove home holding hands. It turned out to be another beautiful day.

The first thing I did with Sandy when we got home was to wheel her out onto the deck. It was a little windy; but I placed the latest toy into her hands--a remote control for the electric awning. In past years, Sandy enjoyed spending as much time as possible out on our deck and now she could control the sun. "Can you feel the power?" she would type on her writing board! "Yes, Arnold", I would reply.

We would pack as much as possible in to every home visit. Weekends were literally filled with many ups and downs!

As a surprise for Sandy, I had a contractor install an over-head lift track just above our outside hot tub. My sister, Diane, and my daughter, Linda, assisted Sandy with putting on a nice bathing suit and wrapped her up in the water resistant body sling that we used to lift her over her bed.

Anxiously awaiting her arrival, I went downstairs and attached the motorized lift. The weather was very cold and I was wondering about the holdup. Perhaps while waiting, I should have had on some proper pants and a warm jacket. (No, I wasn't wearing a Speedo!)

I was completely frozen and ready to give up, just as the ladies appeared all dressed as if they were in the Caribbean and ready to hit the beach. Sandy had several bright striped towels wrapped around her body.

We pushed the wheelchair close to the side of the hot tub and hooked the sling into place. With final instructions for Sandy to keep her hands and arms tucked inside, I engaged the motor. Nothing happened.

I quickly jumped into the steaming water and started fumbling with the controls. Finally I had success! Sandy began to rise like an angel into the sky. Everyone was so excited.

Half way up, it jammed again. Sandy was swinging like a piñata. As panic began setting in, I started splashing hot water on Sandy in an effort to warm her and begin the retreat. Try as I might, it just wouldn't work; so I engaged the safety mode and disengaged the motor while gingerly lowering Sandy into the water. We would obviously have to figure out an exit plan.

We all had a great time doing something that Sandy always enjoyed; but in the back of my mind I knew getting Sandy out, was going to be a challenge.

We stayed in the water until our prune like skin dictated it was time to vacate the hot tub. Getting Sandy back into the house before frostbite set in was tricky. It was worth the effort; but not the risk; so shortly afterwards we sold the hot tub.

༺༻

A New Addition to Our Family

It was October 15, 2008 and I had arranged a surprise for Sandy. Our doorbell rang and one by one the little puppies were scurrying everywhere. Sandy was shocked; but I could tell that she was very excited at what was happening. In total, about six little cockapoos were lifted unto her hydraulic bed located in our dining room. As so often is the case, one little gal made an especially fond attachment to Sandy, and would not leave her side. While the others all scampered about, this puppy pressed hard into Sandy's side and would not leave.

There was no question--*she* had selected *us*. Completely black, with a touch of pure white patch just below the neck, she very quickly made her way into our lives. It's a good thing we bought this puppy when she was tiny because she liked to crawl up and snuggle against Sandy's neck.

We named her Lucy, mostly because we are just not very original; and because the name was easy to say. She quickly became Sandy's girl. The two of them were inseparable and grew extremely close. I had the onerous task of trying to maintain the lawn and keep our condo management people at bay.

Sandy was never really a "dog person"; and she used to get very bored when I told her stories of my earlier days training German Shepherds and Rottweilers at The Alberta Schutzhund Club. In my opinion, this was definitely not a working dog; but in the months that followed, Lucy won over my heart as well.

I recall one particular day when I was not very impressed. The breeder told me that this breed of dog was extremely intelligent and easy to train. All I can tell you is that it was not long before Lucy had me wrapped around her little paw. If I raised my voice when Lucy piddled, Sandy would get upset with me. If

I corrected Lucy from jumping on people, Sandy would give me a strange look as if to say, "So much for the expert dog trainer"; like it was my job or something!

Perhaps I did not pay enough attention to the quirks of this little dog; and didn't appreciate just how much trouble she could get into. When she would tire of destroying the house, she would turn her vengeance onto her long necked rubber chicken. I was glad when the day came that she crushed the squeaking device; at least I no longer had to listen to the high pitched annoying noise. The guy that invented that thing must have had the mind of a criminal. Many nights, Lucy robbed me of a good sleep. Why she felt the urge to attack the chicken at night, was beyond any of my training.

The moment I truly had to wonder about the sanity of this mutt, came one day when we were all stretched out relaxing on top of our bed. Sandy was upright and I was lying facing her. Looking back, it all seems like a really bad dream; but I will never forget what Lucy did next. Without warning, she stood up and headed towards me. I thought she was going to jump off the bed and get her chicken to bug me. Perhaps a game of fetch was about to be happening. I was not to be that lucky; because the next thing I remember was a warm stream of urine pouring onto my face. Sandy broke into hysterical laughter and tears ran down her face...all at my expense. I told her that she had a sick sense of humor; and she just laughed harder.

The dog survived, and I did my best to forget this awful experience. It did, however, change the dynamics of our relationship in a profound way. I do not like small dogs on our bed; and this episode ended a close bond.

I recall wondering if we had made the right decision to take on this added responsibility. Lucy had a mind of her own; and quite a protective personality when it came to Sandy. This dog thought she was a body guard. Sandy used to laugh at Lucy's antics; however, most of the time I was less than amused.

One day everything changed as to how I viewed this little troublemaker. I was downstairs and Sandy was in bed. I was suddenly greeted by Lucy. It was not her normal greeting to which I had become accustomed. This time it was different. She barked incessantly and would run towards the doorway leading upstairs. Quickly returning to me, she started jumping and racing back to the stairs. Clearly she wanted me to follow her.

I began walking upstairs and then I heard it. Sandy was choking! By the time I reached Sandy, she was turning color. I didn't panic; but it did take a while to get Sandy breathing properly again. From this day forward, I would never complain about Lucy again.

When times got tough, and Sandy had the strength, we would go on weekend trips. I recall our going to the Jasper Park Lodge one weekend. We couldn't take Lucy, with us; but because she was such a small dog we had no trouble finding a dog sitter. The lodge provided us with wonderful accommodations and we were situated right on the lake. It was a good thing Lucy was not with us as the elk were in their rut and very aggressive. One bull was right outside our door; and was not very happy. We settled down and enjoyed a long morning coffee in front of our fireplace, but not before I managed to smoke out the entire cabin. Someone should have put a large note instructing would-be outdoorsmen like me to open the damper PRIOR to lighting.

When we did venture out, it began as a stroll and progressed into a running marathon as we dodged the elk and the bitter cold morning air. In hindsight, we should have brought the power wheelchair. We headed for the nearest entrance of the main lodge facilities. We enjoyed a nice warm drink in front of their massive fireplace with no worries about having to control the blaze or the smoke. After a quick trip to the washroom, we were ready to go for a drive around town.

As Sandy's caregiver, washrooms were always a challenge for me. Typically, I would run surveillance and watch the door for a while before entering. With no sounds coming from within its closed doors, we would hustle into the washroom, often taking with us remnants of the door frames. The faster I could get this job done, the better!

I recall saying to Sandy, that this was one sweet washroom! Talk about classy. The routine was generally pretty clear but some facilities are a little cramped. This one was perfect, until we heard the door open and two elderly ladies talking. The sound of their voices quickly came to an end. I suspect they looked down and saw my boots next to Sandy's feet. Normally this would not have been a problem; however this day, Sandy got the giggles.

There we were, in the women's washroom, laughing hysterically. The more I tried to quiet Sandy, the louder her squeals became. I was dying. Obviously this did not look or sound good. The elderly ladies vacated quickly; no doubt looking for the hotel security. We hightailed it out of there and hurried back to our cabin. Not even the elk could keep up with us.

※

Sad Turn of Events

Sadly, Lucy passed away prematurely. Perhaps she knew in some strange way that she had fulfilled her role in Sandy's life. Despite rushing her to a wonderful clinic, her days were over. I remember thinking at the time that it might just be something simple; but the x-rays would reveal otherwise. With leash in hand I returned home...without Sandy's precious little girl.

There was no question that someday we would get another dog; but for now, we just needed to get over our loss. For anyone going through a difficult time in his or her life, we would strongly recommend adopting a pet. Despite the rough start, the joy that Lucy brought us was worth every challenge. Like most things in life, we must never take anything for granted. There are never any guarantees. We will remain eternally grateful for the wonderful memories and the times that we shared with Lucy.

❦

Sandy's Thoughts

I was never a "dog person"--or so I thought; but Lucy was my precious little buddy; and of course she was very therapeutic on all levels. We will definitely get another dog but there would never be another Lucy.

This chapter makes me appreciate just how far I have already come. Not being able to take in anything via mouth was dreadful. The constant dry throat and parched lips drove me nuts; but it was the social aspect that bothered me the most. Of course "failing" any test was unacceptable.

I miss our hot tub; so perhaps we will purchase another one. I will have to insist on something easier to get into though, as the thought of hanging and dangling up in the air like some prized catch of the day while David tries to figure things out, doesn't thrill me.

As for my desire to race around in my power wheelchair I think Dave is exaggerating. My problem is not so much speed...but accuracy. One day, I think I scared him big time! Dave was standing at the top of the stairs leading down to the workout room. Normally I slowly glide up to him, come to a full stop and he assists me out of the chair. Unfortunately, I forgot to shut off the power to the chair and I accidentally hit the fast speed throttle causing me to lurch forward. The chair itself weighs several hundred pounds, and with my added weight you can understand why David might have been concerned.

There was at least an inch before things would have gone south. David is such a worrywart.

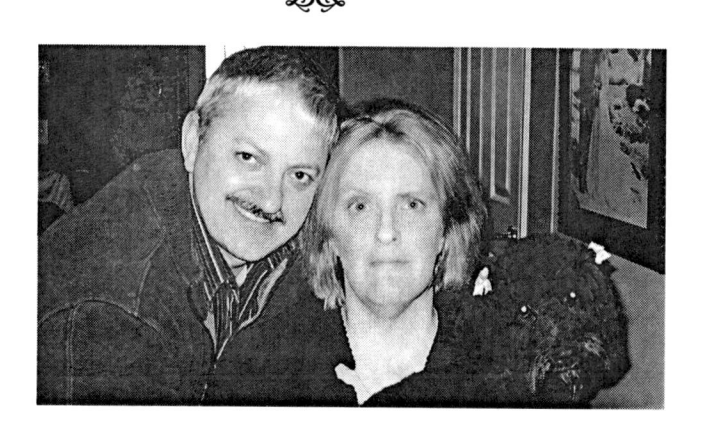

༺༻

OUR LITTLE LUCY...NEVER FORGOTTEN

Chapter Ten

❧

Rebuilding Sandy

Once released from the Glenrose, Sandy would have all the tools she would need to progress on her own. In total, Sandy spent a year in care; six months at the University of Alberta Hospital and five and a half months at the Glenrose Rehabilitation Hospital. We will never forget those days but now it was time to move on and continue this marathon.

With Sandy now surpassing all the expectations and back in her own home, there would be more adventures to come. Sandy was now able to force out some distinguishable words; and she had good muscle strength in her legs--not perfect but workable!

It took a while for us to get connected with the right surgeon; but eventually we would have the good fortune of meeting a doctor by the name of Dr. Angela Scharfenberger. The day was met with a high level of anxiety; but at the same times much anticipation. We had heard that she was the best! "Anything to get rid of these braces"; Sandy would often say! The leopard design print was cool; but with having to tightly secure the many straps while positioning Sandy's feet into position was torture. It was not going to improve with time, unless there was some serious medical reconstruction.

The meeting with Dr. Scharfenberger went well; although the thought of being bedridden once again for a couple of months didn't sit well with Sandy. At least we still had the ceiling lifts in place.

Dr. Scharfenberger was willing to perform what would amount to a life altering step for Sandy. She proposed rebuilding Sandy's legs in an effort to correct the dramatic feet inversions that had occurred as a result of lying in bed for so long.

We had heard that Dr. Angela Scharfenberger has a background in therapy. She, along with another talented surgeon, Dr. S.K. Dulai, would work together on this difficult surgery which would cut the time down that would be needed to complete this delicate operation. They had worked together before and we were confident having met both of them that Sandy would be in good hands. Sandy's lower legs would need to be reconstructed. It would involve lowering her arches, extending her Achilles tendons and grafting various ligaments and tendons to opposite sides of her feet.

We understood that by working side by side, this operation would still take the better part of a day. It would hopefully give Sandy the means to stand upright without her braces and even perhaps take steps. They were confident that once things healed, after about two to three months, Sandy's ankles and feet would be able to bear weight. The defining moment would be when the casts would eventually come off; and Sandy would walk again!

Prior to this incredible surgery, it was impossible for Sandy to stand for more than about a second or two; therefore, the decision was not that difficult. Of course this was easy for me to say; I wasn't the one who would have to handle going through all of the grief.

As mentioned before, following Sandy's surgery, she would be completely bedridden, again. There would be several cast changes. While this was being done, I passed the time trying to count the hundreds of stitches and staples now visible for my viewing pleasure—at least the ones that I could see. I remember the feeling of almost passing out and having to repeatedly collect myself. It shocked me that she was not suffering much pain—especially considering all that had been done.

I will never forget the day, many months later, when we returned to the hospital to have Dr. Scharfenberger witness Sandy take a few steps. We had not brought along her walker, but we had been practising; so we were ready to impress. We improvised by Sandy pushing me in her wheelchair! Sandy's surgeon was so delighted, and shared in our special moment! Unfortunately Dr. Dulai was busy attending to another patient upstairs so we did not get a chance to thank her personally as well; but some day we hope to pay her a visit. What they accomplished together was nothing short of another miracle. Indeed, the days ahead were starting to look a little brighter.

Immediately following this difficult surgery, they tried feeding Sandy some soft food. Sandy, still affected by the drugs, didn't tell them she could not swallow. Trying to feed Sandy this soon was a BIG mistake! Once again, Sandy ended up in ICU. By this time we were getting to know everyone there on a first name basis. "Sandy is back to visit us", they would say. Fortunately they suctioned everything and once again, a crisis was averted.

It was during this time of recovery, that Sandy received the following note from one of our caregivers, my eldest daughter, Linda.

It read:

Dear Sandy,

In the pain and in the dark there is always a light.
My light, in the darkness is Sandra Nette and experiencing our own special relationship. The new growth of a beautiful friendship and an endless amount of laughs you bring to my day. Rest assured honey, with your change you are changing people!

I know we want the old you back, but I love the new you! I admire your courage and spirit, your tears even your cries. That's just part of life and we will embrace it with you. Your sense of humour and resolve are a testament of who you are and what we all can be.

I know you've changed me and brought new meaning to my life. You've taught me how to harness my inner strength, given me a serious lesson in patience. And for these things alone Sandy I thank you.

Just remember this work within you is not completed. There will be many more miracles to come even if you do not recognize them at first. I'm just glad to be a part of your life.

Ultimately, the operation on rebuilding Sandy's legs was a success. Today, not only can Sandy walk with a walker, but with the use of hand rails in our home and with guidance make it up the stairs to our master bedroom.

⚜

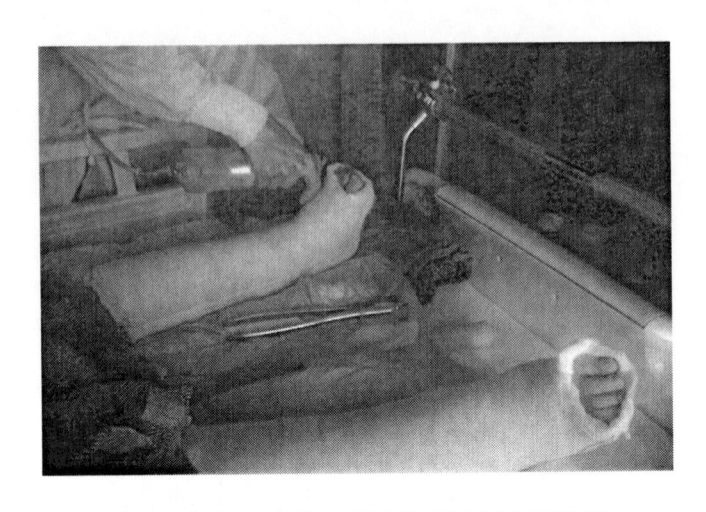

BEDRIDDEN AGAIN BUT ALL WORTH IT

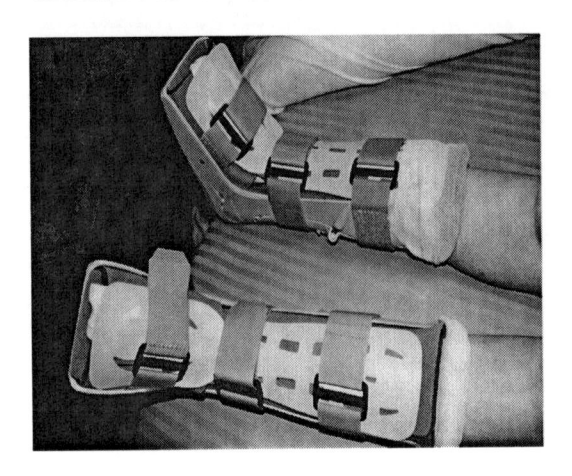

NICE BOOTS SANDY

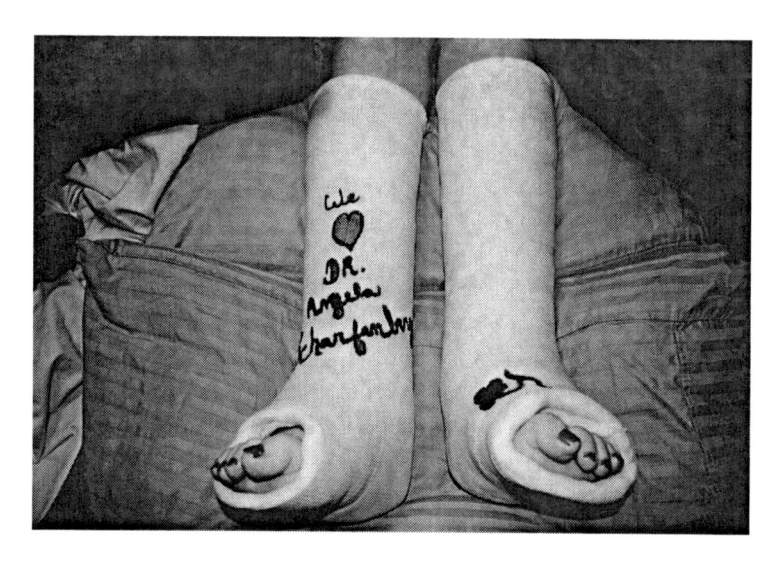

DAVID TOOK GOOD CARE OF MY TOES

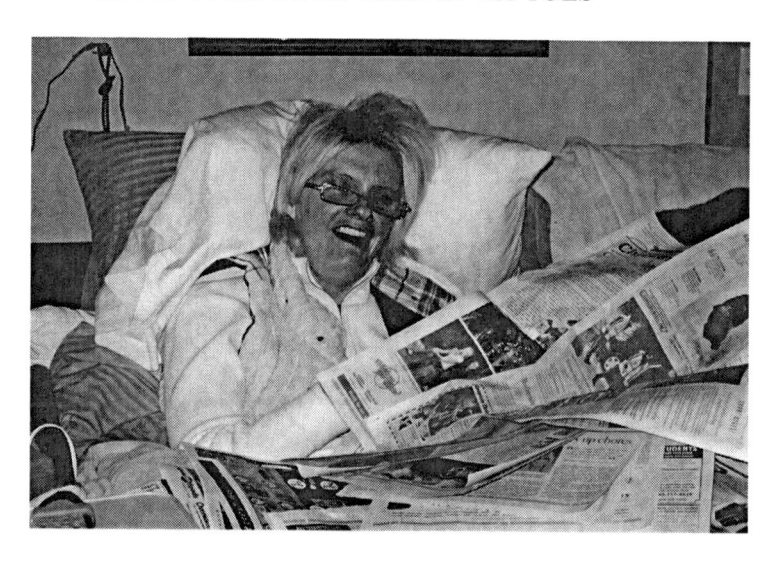

*STUCK BACK IN BED AGAIN BUT AT LEAST I AM
GETTING CAUGHT UP WITH MY READING*

Hidden Tears

It was hard to believe, but it was already February 2009. I was having trouble sleeping that night. The day was somewhat of an emotional period.

Sandy had outpatient therapy that afternoon; something she looked forward to every day. Sandy was coming along with her speech therapy as well, and could verbalize three or four words. These achievements take enormous effort and concentration on her part. Given all of these positive things, I'm not exactly sure what came over me that day.

It started with a simple shower. While I prepared Sandy I suddenly began to weep. I quickly reached in and turned on the taps hoping the sound of the rushing water would drown out what was happening. I thought I had this under control.

As mentioned earlier, for those who know me most would agree that I wear my heart on my sleeve. I constantly try to control my emotions, trying to focus only on the positive. This day, however, there was to be no such luck.

Eventually it was impossible to hide the flood of tears, and Sandy soon realized exactly what was happening. She reached up and I bent over as Sandy pulled me closer and wrapped her hands around my neck. "Everything's gonna be okay", she would reassure me. "Just hang in there, Dave."

I managed to pull myself together and transferred her to the shower chair without dropping her. I truly appreciated the shower that day because I was able to stand behind Sandy and resume my tears knowing she would be none the wiser. You have to be creative sometimes. After a while I was able to collect myself and bring these wayward emotions under control.

Sandy had come such a long way; yet both of us still realized the enormous challenges that remained before us. As a couple, so much had changed. In many ways we accepted the painstakingly slow path to recovery; but we were always hopeful that Sandy would regain a full life. At other times, it would just get the better of us; therefore, the occasional meltdown.

Don't get me wrong friends; the good times are still there for us as a couple, and more powerful than ever. Sandy laughs almost daily at all of the crazy things that seem to follow us; like some twisted joke at times. We still continue to grow as a married couple; sometimes disagreeing with each other, although not very often. Sometimes we're just silent.

Then there are days when one or both of us lose it. Mostly, we appreciate each other; and accept that we're not in control of what happens down the road. I guess it's just the suddenness of everything that sometimes happens in life which seems to shock you into a different zone of existence. For a while we felt like we were outside ourselves.

Getting used to this type of relationship intensity on a daily basis, takes some mental adjustment. I mostly know what Sandy is thinking before she speaks; and when I don't clue in, she looks at me like I just failed the first grade. I absolutely love her sense of humour!

Tornado

A few months later, on a very hot July evening, after spending the day with Sandy's big brother, Dave, and his lovely wife, Lynn, we were heading back to Edmonton when we noticed that the weather appeared to be turning nasty. As I don't like driving in the dark at the best of times, we decided not to stop for a bite to eat and just hurry home. It always takes us a while to get Sandy through her nightly routine and ready for bed; so we didn't want to be too late getting home.

The day had been so much fun. I will never forget when our unannounced arrival was met with strange stares. Sandy had gotten her blond hair dyed dark brown, and they had not seen her new look. After the confusion ended, they rushed to greet us to their special part of the world.

They have a lovely secluded spot deeply tucked away in the trees, which provided much needed shade that day. We appreciated their location, as Sandy must take extreme care on the amount of sun she gets because the meds cause skin sensitivity. We went around the resort and met many of their wonderful friends.

By the time we reached Edmonton, the weather appeared to be calming down. Ever since Black Friday, the day of Edmonton's devastating tornado, whenever the sky turns ugly, many of Edmonton's residents notice and have become very wary. We remember Black Friday because people lost their lives and the memories are etched in our minds.

I got Sandy ready for bed and noticed that her legs had swollen considerably over the course of the day. Perhaps it was from the heat. She was so relieved when her braces came off. I raised the bed and prepared her suction pump along with her nightly medication.

As I was gathering things for the night, I glanced out our large window which overlooks the North Saskatchewan River and the open fields below. We have an almost perfect 180 degree commanding view for many miles. There was an eerie feeling as a massive storm front quickly began to form around us. Like a huge dark series of clouds all banding together, the formation began to roll. In what seemed like just minutes, the clouds began to break open and down came the rain...in buckets! The water was rushing into our garage as the hail filled our water grate in seconds. The rain was relentless. I couldn't believe what I was seeing! All I could think was...what next...locusts?

I pulled Sandy up and showed her what was happening. I knew things might get worse and didn't want to cause excess worry; so I tried not to show Sandy too much of my increasing panic. We would have to get dressed again, and hurry down to the basement. This was no easy task at this time of night!

With marathon speed, I put Sandy's sweats on her and finished getting her dressed. I put her braces back on in record time despite the tight fit. Needless to say, my wife was very impressed. This was called my turbo mode.

By this time, the thunder was beginning to build; and a huge wind raced through our home sounding like a locomotive. We retreated to Sandy's built-in shower; because this would be the safest place to hide. It was reinforced and situated in our basement. There are no windows in there; and we were within earshot of our van's radio which I had left turned on for emergency updates. With extra water and a blanket we were ready.

While I was briefly upstairs, I witnessed our neighbour's new steel gazebo twist like a pretzel. This would be no ordinary storm; I thought to myself.

We used the interior shelves of the shower to hold our various last minute emergency supplies. Then we sat there feeling a little foolish. One must prepare for these types of emergencies; especially when extra time is needed to get ready. We enjoyed a nice supper; even though it was a little crowded. I think we will come up with a better hiding place for the next time Mother Nature takes a swing.

We eventually made it back up to bed that night; but I was covered in sweat by the time all was said and done. At least I didn't have to go far for the shower.

The next day, we went for a drive around Edmonton to survey the damage caused by this storm. Although not officially classified as a tornado, the damage was everywhere. Thousands of trees were damaged, road signs smashed to bits, roofs damaged, industrial buildings collapsed, and even serious damage to our CN Tower located downtown. Driving along, we also saw a semi-trailer on its side, and many cars damaged from large hail stones. Fortunately, no one was injured and we didn't have a repeat of July 31, 1987.

❧

Lights Out

I checked on Sandy and she was fast asleep. I normally catch her before she dozes off, and we do our nightly routine. I didn't want to wake her from a sound sleep; but I went ahead and rubbed some special fragrant lotion on her face and little hands. This is a ritual that I adopted and Sandy doesn't seem to mind. I caught a faint smile, and then she went back to sleep. We have both come to appreciate this time of day so much. Sleep, and the dreams that follow, are a means of escape for Sandy--a time when she could be normal again; to finish her piano piece, sing a song, go for a walk or chase me around the house. Often by morning, it would take Sandy a while to comprehend that she just couldn't jump up and get out of bed.

Mornings came early, and it was getting increasingly more difficult for me to go to work. Sometimes just answering the phone was a challenge; and I feared I was doing my clients a disservice. I could not seem to stay focused or concentrate on anything work related. Sandy was my priority; and getting her better was all I could think about at that moment. My memory was never great; and at this point I wasn't sure what I should call it. I was thinking that I was too young to be experiencing dementia; although I had aged considerably right before my eyes.

Looking back, I was once accused of putting Sandy at the center of my universe. I couldn't believe the comment at the time; but I do understand why one might have thought this was somehow not the best. This was during a time when Sandy was fully dependent 24/7 on the help around her; when she could choke to death at any minute on her our own vomit. For me, there was never any question as to where Sandy must be in my world!

This came from someone who loved her, and I'm sure it was well meant, but it cut to the core. Definitely one of those times when I would cry out "forgive them Lord; they know not what they say".

I desperately wanted to try to understand why such words would ever be spoken. Sandy *was* the center of my universe; and my world had to rotate around her. I wanted to meet her needs; not because of a sense of duty, but out of love and compassion.

Some things would never make sense. We have to move forward and just leave it at that.

Sandy's Thoughts

Coming home was magical. Even though I had enjoyed some weekend home retreats previously, this was permanent. Deep down I knew that we could at least start living a more normal life even though the finish line remained nowhere in sight.

My needs were still substantial but my caregivers were tremendous. David was patient and always very supportive. I truly had a great team and never once did I feel like I was suffering in silence anymore; actually it was quite the opposite....if I was having a bad day, everyone knew about it!

Crammed into the downstairs stairwell landing, I was forced to listen to Dave tell me how he was going to build a cement bomb shelter. Okay...maybe I am exaggerating this time; but I think my husband wanted to prepare for just about anything. It's as though he has a protective shield around me...and I love it!

The visit to my brother's and sister-in-law's lake resort was very special and just like old times. I would tease my brother and when he bent down to get in for a group photo I'd pinch his nose. He was always such a laid back good sport about all of my antics and was accustomed to my giving him the what for! We have a unique relationship and I will never forget the day my husband met my "little" former football player brother. I think David was expecting a much smaller framed man as I was so slim and small boned. All my hubby kept saying was "good grief Sandy...how is this even possible"?

With each passing month I am becoming more and more aware of this new mind of mine. It's weird not to feel the fear or the anxiety anymore. It was second nature before my stroke and now worry was becoming just a minor irritant --and that I CAN HANDLE!

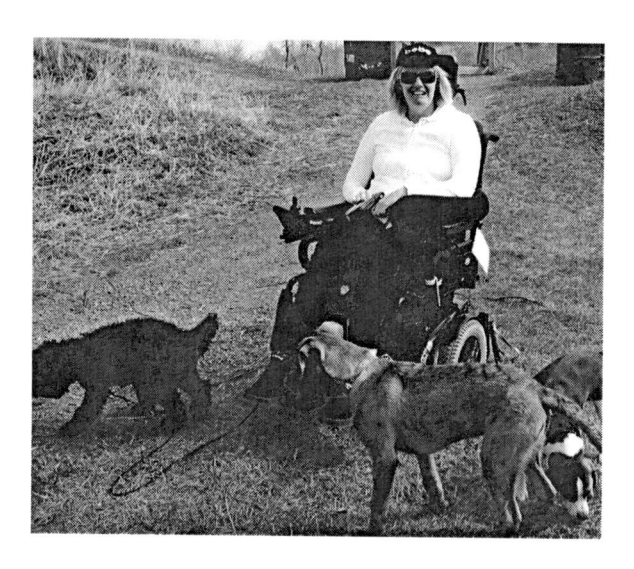

NO DAVID, YOU CAN'T USE MY CHAIR TO WALK THE DOG

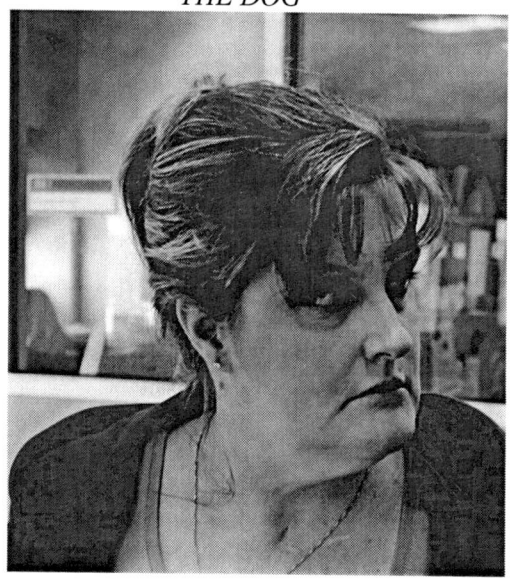

WORKING OUT AT THE CRIS CLINIC

Chapter Eleven

❧❧

Jaw Dropping

It was now 2012. We received the long anticipated call from Dr. Walter Dobrovolsky. This incredible surgeon was ready to rebuild Sandy's jaw, consequently enabling future restorative plastic surgery that would improve her ability to speak. It would be one of the most painful procedures that Sandy endured; but with huge benefits to come.

Following the surgery, Sandy, as you can tell by the picture, looked like a plane crash survivor; but just as the doctor promised, her jaw opening improved with each passing month. We have the utmost respect for this talented surgeon and consider our meeting him to be a huge blessing. We would, once again call it the Alberta Advantage!

This was paving the way for Sandy's final operation which is her throat reconstruction. A plastic surgeon would perform this next intricate operation in the coming months; and hopefully as a result, Sandy would regain some of her ability to speak and be understood. Presently when she "talked" it depleted all of her air supply; just like a balloon emptying. Even the fact that she could speak at all, was a miracle. Her throat had apparently developed a muscle that protruded enough to enhance pressure against her vocal chords. The human body is indeed an amazing thing!

In the past, Sandy loved to sing, and she had a great voice. If I pressed her she would play the piano and sing for me; but rarely for an audience. Her voice truly was as sweet as you could imagine. It will be very interesting to hear what she sounds like after her upcoming throat operation. We are hopeful that once completed, Sandy will have more volume and not be so easily winded when attempting to speak or to be heard.

※

Reflection

Without this intense degree of personal suffering, Sandy's life would most likely have remained pretty much in the same place. She used to struggle with anxiety, and to some degree a condition called Obsessive Compulsive Disorder (OCD). Long past are those distant memories of her wanting and feeling the need, to solve the world's problems on her own; and of trying to "measure up", despite having achieved excellent job status and career satisfaction.

Things happened during her hospital stays and long afterwards. Some of these things would defy any possible explanation.

The fact that Sandy no longer required any medication for anxiety or her obsessive compulsive nature was truly a blessing. This was indeed, a miracle; although an unexpected one. Even for someone without these struggles, I could not imagine for one moment, her having gone through something as serious as Locked-in Syndrome and not going completely crazy.

Sandy saw a picture of a lady whose face and hands had literally been ripped and bitten off by a chimpanzee gone wild. The victim was recently told that after a long battle with trying to save what they could, the doctors would have to remove her eyes. There was a single photo of her covering up, trying to conceal herself, so as not to alarm others. Expressing this woman's vulnerability to the world provoked thoughts of our own situation.

You will always find someone else worse off than yourself; so there is really no point in complaining. Being pushed around in a wheelchair through malls, and stared at by the public would no longer have quite the same impact. It was time to take these lemons and make some lemonade.

It's been over five years since her stroke and Sandy's speech continues to improve. Even the ability to open her mouth wider has helped with the volume. Not long ago, on a day pass, I took Sandy to the movie theater. She motored herself to the ice cream vendor, while I attempted to get some popcorn to satisfy my own addiction.

Sandy made her way up the line but apparently encountered some trouble once she had reached the counter. The young man tending the till thought she needed Kleenex. He made this astute assumption based on the observation that Sandy was plugging her nose while talking to him and trying to place her order. With her nostrils closed, Sandy was able to prevent air from escaping, thus projecting sound better; however, this time it didn't work.

I hustled Sandy into the pitch black theater, almost pushing her over the edge and down some stairs. Sandy was freaking out; but I told her I had seen the edge at the last second and not to worry. We fumbled our way to the handicapped section, ran over a few feet and settled down to enjoy the show. "Not so fast" Sandy said. "I still want my ice cream!"

I ran back to get her the ice cream, and thanked the young lad for at least trying to understand what Sandy had requested. I was thinking that at least we had made it to the theater; and this was progress in its own right!

We weren't as fortunate the last time we tried going to the movies. The theaters were located on the third floor and we had to use several different elevators to get there. We had quickly rushed to arrive on time, and when we finally arrived, despite the theaters now within plain view, the last elevator was unfortunately out of service.

We complained to each other; but realizing there were no options, we turned around and started heading back to our vehicle.

As we were returning to the van, there was a fire alarm. That was another interesting experience all on its own. People were running, vendors were rolling down their shutters and an entire downtown shopping mall turned into a ghost town right before our eyes.

As a matter of fire safety, the second set of elevators which we had used to get up to the main level shut down. No problem. A passing security guard advised us to use the freight elevator to our left, just through some nearby exit doors. We did this...I mean we tried to do this.

About fifteen long minutes passed; and we remained in front of the large elevator doors. The elevator never arrived so we decided to go back to the main area and ask someone else for assistance. There was just one problem; there was no one in sight. Elvis had left the building. Can you say "feeling vulnerable"?

We waited for the fire department while we listened to the commands coming over the loud P.A. system. "Do not use the elevators or escalators. Use the stairs only; and leave through the nearest exit immediately." We couldn't use the escalator if we tried. What a predicament!

After what seemed like an eternity, the alarms ceased; and at least we were able to think. A fellow carrying a ladder rushed by us, and said to hang in there! He assured us that the elevators would be up and running soon. We didn't smell any smoke; so we decided to trust this guy. He was right. No sooner had he left us, and the elevators were running once again. We hurried into the working elevators, and both let out a huge sigh of relief.

Providing that we ever wanted to try this again, we decided that we would stick to ground level theaters.

୭୬୨୦

Bad Hair Day

It had been a few days since our theater escapade, and wanting to make up for the fiasco, I decided to impress Sandy. The day was beautiful; therefore, I figured it was time to get Sandy outside for some fresh air. No caregivers were available; but I knew that I could handle things on my own.

I wheeled Sandy over to the table, brought out her make-up and ran upstairs to get my laptop.

Sandy looked at me in a strange manner, and asked what I was going to do with the computer. I told her to relax; and that I had everything under control. Her job was to just sit back and take it easy.

I am kind of a hands-on guy who is not afraid to tackle anything…or so I thought. On the web, I looked up *How To French Braid.* Sandy began to sweat.

The next couple of hours dragged on and on and on. Sandy's scalp ached from the constant pulling and redoing. Over and over I would ask for just one more chance to get it right. She was such a good sport.

The gal on the computer screen made this look like a cakewalk. Eventually much to Sandy's delight my computer battery went dead. She ended up with a tight ponytail on which I had used a can of hair spray. I also did some magnificent backcombing that I had seen the caregivers do. I decided to leave the French braiding to the experts. This was well above my pay grade; and any hope that I ever had of becoming a hairdresser had been effectively terminated.

However, we weren't finished; next came the makeup. I figured that this would be a cinch, as I have a lot of artistic skills touching up furniture and mixing colours. Unfortunately my ability to refinish furniture would provide Sandy little in the way of comfort. Upon completing her makeup, I wheeled her in front of a large mirror. This was not a good idea. I removed the makeup and reapplied it over and over and over again. Eventually I mastered this art of putting makeup on Sandy. At least she no longer looked like she was applying for a job with the circus.

※

I'm Not Perfect Either Dave

In the following weeks, Sandy made a real effort to make me feel appreciated and reminded me that she was not perfect either. I think she saw that I was frustrated with my limitations in being able to help her.

One day, she came flying into the living room in high gear following a big push from her caregiver, my sister, Diane. As Sandy passed by me, she raised both arms high into the air and yelled out as best as she could, "look mom...no hands!"

It broke the mood; and once again we laughed our way into a better headspace. My wife was never one to shy away from the uncomfortable; and encouraged me to tell Diane the story about the time Sandy almost killed me--okay, maybe not quite an attempt on my life that night; but very interesting just the same.

It went something like this. Sandy and I were dating and in the early stages of getting to know each other. For the most part, Sandy would come over to my place and I would fix us a nice romantic meal. I loved to cook and found it relaxing; so I didn't mind this role reversal. However, one night was to be different. Sandy came over with a beautiful large fillet of wild salmon, fresh asparagus, rice and all the trimmings. She instructed me to go into the living room, put my feet up and watch TV. I was to relax and leave everything to Sandy. I thought, "what a sweetheart"!

This was quite the change, as Sandy had always admitted to me that she was not an experienced cook. Her preference was to dine out in the best restaurants, every day if she had her way!

As I sat in the living room, I remember feeling so grateful that Sandy would come over after already working a full day, and want to please me. The smell was wonderful and I was starving.

Suddenly I heard Sandy let out a gasp. She was very upset and sounded extremely agitated so I got up and wandered into the kitchen. She had apparently forgotten to remove the gauze under the fish prior to putting it into the pan. The plastic and cotton filling had melted into the fish.

She was visibly ticked off and very sad that she had forgotten this minor step. I assured Sandy that it would be fine, providing she scraped off the bottom of the fish. She refused to eat a single bite and said I was crazy. I told her that this was too much money to waste and it tasted great!

I continued devouring the meal until suddenly I got a strange taste in my mouth. It was nothing that a little soya sauce couldn't cure.

Sandy could not believe that I was actually enjoying this meal. She wondered if she had made a mistake by throwing hers into the garbage.

The rest of the night was pretty much a blur. I do remember the sudden onset of extreme stomach cramping and crawling on the floor. I was sweating profusely and my temperature spiking. I finally had to concede and tell Sandy to call my brother-in-law, Nico, who fortunately lived nearby. If we could not have reached him, the only other solution would have been to call an ambulance, as I could not walk on my own. Perhaps I waited too long.

As Sandy will attest, I have no tolerance for pain. Once in the emergency ward, people quickly cleared a path. Perhaps the vomit spraying all over the walls had something to do with it; and the response time from the nurses was excellent. They had me into my own little cubicle in no time.

I didn't really know Sandy very well. However, I recall her sitting in the corner of the room watching as I writhed in pain. My ass was sticking up toward the ceiling and my hands were trying to bend the metal bed rails.

Two Demerol shots in the rear and I was starting to settle down. I looked at Sandy who was sporting several enormous cold sores. They apparently popped out when Sandy saw two uniformed police officers standing just outside my curtain. Sandy later told me that she was worried they would ask her why she did not partake of the meal she had so carefully prepared for us. Sandy thought she would be charged with murder!

Since I am writing this book, obviously I survived. However, for the most part, I take care of the cooking when Sandy and I are alone. It's just safer.

Sandy's Thoughts

David, David, David…when are you going to quit reminding me of the salmon disaster? Don't you get it? This was just a ploy to make sure that YOU would do all of the cooking! I don't do ironing and I don't do cooking. Never did…never will, Honey.

David's Thoughts

Sandy, Sandy, Sandy…I think we need to talk.

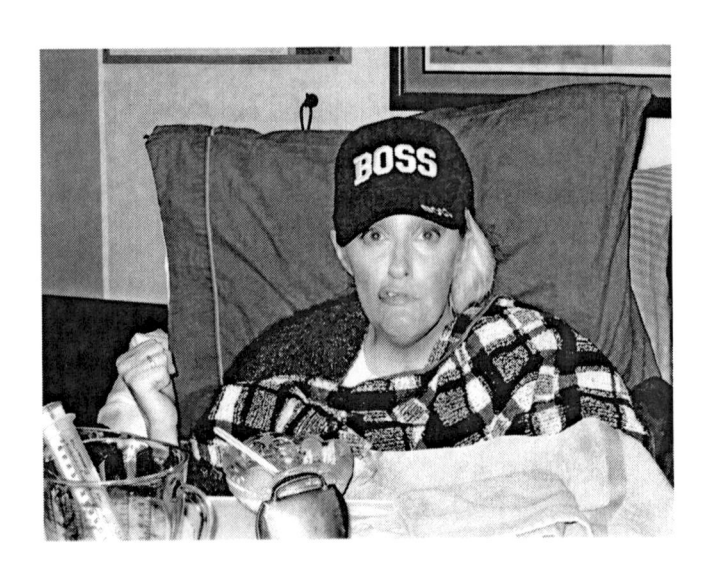

ೊಲ

THE INTIMIDATION LOOK

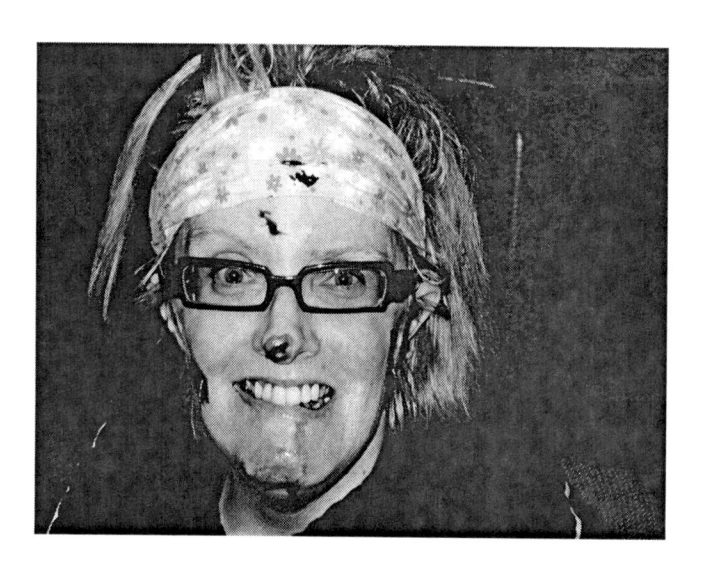

FINE DINING ETIQUETTE

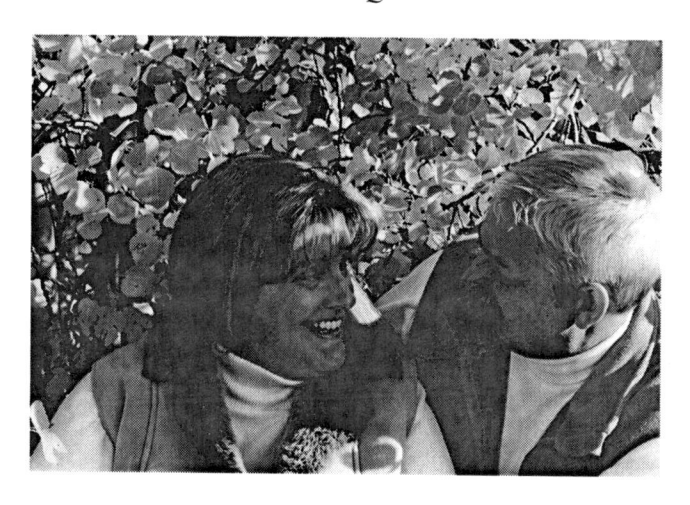

THE FALL...STILL OUR FAVORITE TIME OF YEAR

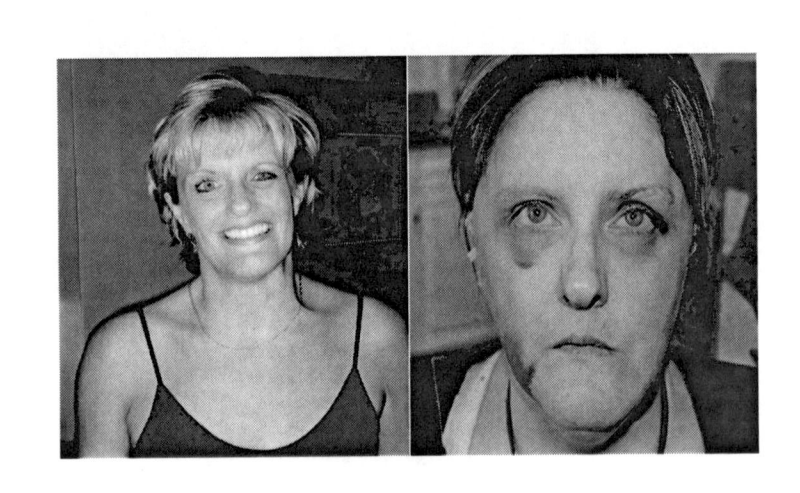

SOMETIMES THE PICTURES SAY IT ALL!

Chapter Twelve

Forged Consent

I will never forget the day.

Just as we were about to go to the door, our lawyer called saying he had some interesting news for us--a change in the defendant's position with respect to a record he produced.

Apparently there were falsified documents that had been submitted to the court when we had tried initially to bring about a class action suit. A signed official document, which would change the course of our destiny. To make a long story short, the chiropractor, who was the defendant, blamed with injuring Sandy, was apparently admitting, under oath, that he lied and committed forgery. Not only was the formal consent document forged, but an admission was also given to falsifying her medical files.

Sandy had always maintained from the very beginning, that what was produced to us was not her signature on the consent form. When initially asked about the consent form, Sandy had expressed to both me and to our lawyer that something was not right with her signature. She did not recognize it. And she certainly did not recall ever signing such a document; nor had she ever been informed of the dangers and possible side effects from an upper neck manipulation.

For Sandy, seeing her chiropractor on a regular basis, was just something everyone, she was told, should do in order to maintain good health. It was a type of maintenance program or so she thought.

At the time, our lawyers indicated that it didn't make sense to accuse the chiropractor of what would essentially be fraud on his part. A criminal offence punishable by possibly years in prison--up to fourteen to be exact we were advised. And how could we prove this? Our legal team was convinced that we had enough of a solid case and we were told that it was probably not even necessary to bring this into the mix.

In the end, we did hire a forensic examiner to inspect the documents in discussion, and as suspected, all were verified to concur with the admissions.

While we cannot discuss the terms of our agreement, nor the exact settlement arrangements, we can say that our case has been settled out of court, and all parties are satisfied.

Questions, however, still remain unanswered. Mainly, why is the practice of rapid upper neck manipulation still allowed to continue even after years of many medical and scientific inquiries have proven it has no medical value? This opinion is not only shared by us, but by many others with whom we have personally spoken.

We've spoken with young men who've lost their livelihoods, mothers who've lost their daughters, people whose lives have been totally wrecked, all as a result of receiving an upper neck manipulation. Some chiropractors have made reference to this practice as "The Hole in One Theory"; and encourage its use from the cradle to the grave, expressing its merits of ridiculous claims.

Fortunately, today, there are fewer and fewer chiropractors utilizing this rapid upper neck twisting "technique". Of the chiropractors who do not engage in this risky procedure estimates range somewhere around the twenty per cent mark. That still leaves the majority still accepting this as a good form of ongoing treatment.

Of course, with all of the publicity from Sandy's case, fewer folks are subjecting themselves to this archaic and dangerous practice. I do not think Sandy will ever become a Poster Child for endorsing any of the so called "benefits" of upper neck twisting. Just one look at any before and after picture of Sandy would stop most logical people in their tracks and make them think twice about having this procedure done at all. In total there are over twenty different types of strokes and all can cause various degrees of disability or death.

Naturally, the more I read and investigated on my own, the more I asked myself how it was that Sandy, in perfect health, paid for a procedure that had such a bad track record in my opinion. Clearly, when the risks of any such action exceed that of any gain, perceived or not, the choice should always be to refrain and consider other options. This, at the very least, should be explained to the patient.

Here in Alberta, we wrote to our members of parliament demanding that they reconsider paying and subsidizing chiropractic treatment at the taxpayers' expense. We were delighted when Alberta followed suit with the majority of other provinces in Canada and delisted chiropractic as a beneficial health service. We perceived this as future lives being saved from harm or worse.

Most of you will be thinking we're totally opposed to chiropractic; but this couldn't be further from the truth. Ever since Sandy's catastrophic injury, our goal has been that they, themselves, as a chiropractic community, would simply look at the numbers of injured people and discontinue their practice of this one single portion of what they do--the rapid upper neck manipulation.

I personally spoke with a neurologist in Edmonton, Alberta, Canada, who has gone on record stating that he has never met a colleague in his field, who has not had at least one victim from a chiropractic session gone wrong. Surely, one would think this speaks volumes; yet the practice continues to this day even after many out of court settlements.

Public documents will bear out that the chiropractor who injured my wife, was handed down a three month suspension, and was told that he would no longer be insured through the CCPA, the Canadian Chiropractic Protection Agency. To this we have no comment.

We are getting on with our lives the best that we can, and are looking forward to Sandy's final operation, her throat reconstruction.

The burning question was always, why did this have to happen in the first place? It all seems so unbelievably tragic that something so unnecessary had to happen at all.

Sandy was not only dealing with the physical challenges, but she felt betrayed by someone she had come to trust. We forgive this chiropractor and hold no animosity or anger. Any bitterness we once experienced has been overshadowed by our desire to just move on. Life is way too short.

Everyone makes mistakes from time to time; it's just that this one really hurt. There's an old saying and we stick by it, "let he who is without sin cast the first stone".

There are some doctors behind the scenes who went well beyond the call of duty. Not a day goes by when we do not think of the kindness and helpful direction they all provided; for the information on the dangers of neck manipulation that was passed along; for sharing the wisdom of their own experiences with this delicate subject and for the day to day guidance they provided.

They made our journey a little easier to maneuver and as a result we escaped many of the pitfalls that previous victims did not have the luxury of avoiding. We would especially like to thank Murray for all of his valuable assistance!

When we use the title "*Doctor*", we use it in the highest respect possible, when referring to our MD's. Chiropractors use this title to give their career choice, power and influence; to exude a level of trust between the patient and themselves. We understand that apparently while in school, they spend a great deal of time perfecting the art of marketing their trade. It's a shame they don't spend as much time studying the human body in an actual certified hospital setting, much like a medical intern, before calling himself or herself "Doctor".

This is still a major thorn in our sides; the idea that they would be able to call themselves "doctors". We are taught from a very young age, to trust our doctor. One lawyer accurately commented that 'chiropractors for the most part simply parade themselves to the public in white coats, masquerading behind the cloaks of deception'. We know this so aptly describes what is still happening today; but will it ever change? We certainly hope so; because we would not wish our worst enemy to go through one day of suffering that Sandy had to endure.

The constant running of the trachea hose down her throat and suctioning just to keep her breathing, ultimately deprived Sandy of much sleep, leading to even more health issues. There are few among us who could handle this aspect of her recovery process and still hang on to hope. While enduring all of this, we would also continuously wonder, if this was to be our last day on earth.

Sandy's Thoughts

This is definitely one of the most difficult chapters for me to share my inner thoughts. Suffice it to say that I have no choice but to accept what has happened and continue to focus on getting better.

I will say, that like my husband David, we both believe there is a reason for everything that happens in life and we are determined never to stop looking for answers to the question... WHY?

Sorry, that's all I have.

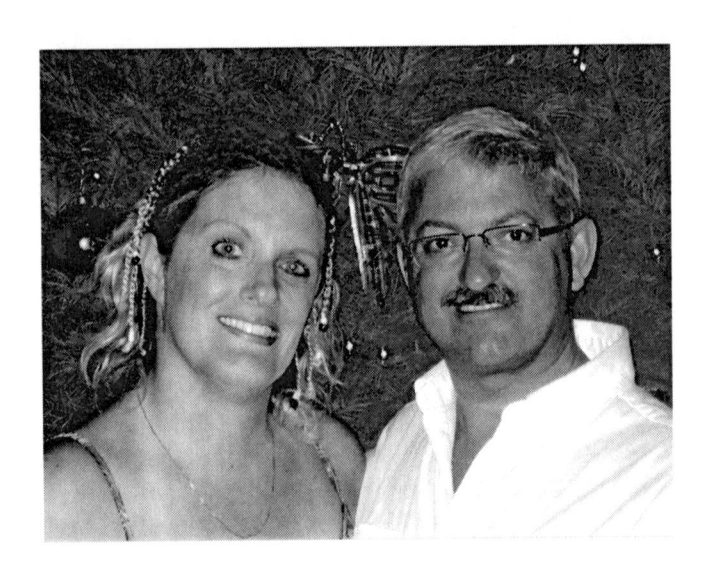

PAST WINTER GET AWAY'S....MY ISLAND GIRL

Chapter Thirteen

The Freight Train

While we were going through these difficult days, we had a lot of time to try and figure out what was at the core of understanding the root of the problem and why nothing appeared to be changing within the wacky world of chiropractic.

When we think of the human species we equate this to our bodies. The human body functions in harmony and there are laws in place which dictate how each part operates. We may vary in blood type, in size, weight, color and shape; but our bodies all operate pretty much the same. Modern medical technologies have presented us with the means of a clearer and defined understanding of how things work.

We know that it is scientifically proven that the nervous system does not "control everything". It doesn't take a brain surgeon to figure out that twisting one's neck, just to hear a popping sound, should play any role in promoting good health. Yet this philosophy continues.

The question remains, why are so many chiropractors claiming that patients need to come in on a regular basis to have these supposed vertebral upper neck subluxations removed? What are subluxations? Chiropractors appear to have their own interpretation of what it is, but it's actually a medical term. In my quest for answers I discovered that their perception is totally different and could best be described as a mystical unseen phantom. It is a condition that apparently cannot be x-rayed or given by the repeated treatments so often prescribed, even corrected for any long term.

Years ago I remember reading about the term subluxation used by a local chiropractor. It certainly sounded official and had a medical flare to it. Apparently these subluxations were even causing people hemorrhoids. Don't laugh....it's true.

In the scientific medical community the term refers to something that does exist. It is defined as two joints that are slightly displaced. The key, however, is in understanding that this almost ALWAYS involves the major joints of our body--NOT the spinal column.

Chiropractors make some big leaps here. They say that they can feel "vertebral subluxations" and that they are typically located in the upper neck area. They boast that they, alone, can do this with their trained hands. No diagnostic tools necessary because nothing would show up on any x-ray. As a result, many chiropractors have long term patients who continue to have their necks manipulated to supposedly correct this defect.

Let's get real. The use of the bare hands to realign vertebrae that are supposedly "subluxated" is a joke. The problem is that if you take this neck twisting procedure away from the majority of chiropractors who still engage in this barbaric upper neck rotation, they become therapists or massage therapists with no special powers. And the need to visit them on a regular basis for ever and ever becomes extinct.

In fact, some have claimed that with only the use of their skilled bare hands, they can feel these imaginary manifestations and therefore, only they can help. In the past, some have even boasted on the web as being able to address everything from bed wetting to cancer. Still other claims being circulated, state that chiropractors can identify over 200 different symptoms and illnesses.

Medical doctors have an obligation as professionals to provide the highest quality of diagnosis and treatment no matter what their field of expertise. The bottom line is that all health care providers, and this includes chiropractors, must base what they do on science, and not some harebrained philosophy. Anything short of science based reasoning would mean there is no standard of care. Could we be onto something?

My wife was subjected to a readjustment of her vertebrae over and over again without any evidence that they had ever been out of place. Sandy was exposed to the highest neck manipulation procedure without any need for it. There is absolutely no benefit for a rapid upper neck manipulation when there is no benefit, and only the risk of permanent injury or even death. Sandy never even complained of getting headaches!

The use of one's hands to realign vertebrae that are supposedly causing subluxations is a false and ridiculous concept from the start. That is not to say that gently massaging one's neck might provide some minor relief to the muscles in this area. Seeing a massage therapist for this and adding some soft music and a steam shower would work as well.

One could go on and on about all the ridiculous methods and so called diagnostic machines that are utilized by this group; but suffice it to say that most of the devices used in assisting with diagnosing nerve dysfunction are simply gimmicks. I had to laugh when I went to a chiropractor and he snapped his fingers along my spine. I thought he was keeping time to the music playing in the background. They get schooling for this type of treatment?

Sandy, an identical twin, was a picture of good health. There was no diabetes in her family, and she had an abundance of energy, often leaving me in the dust. I was not surprised when, through the course of a multitude of daily tests and x-rays, medical personnel would tell me that Sandy was in the best of shape.

On a positive note, we live in an age of rapid communication and there is a thirst for knowledge. People in general, are taking their health into their own hands and realizing the importance of seeking out as much information as possible on any health topic. It's often only a click away; but naturally we must all do our due diligence. Had we searched out chiropractic treatment on Google, regarding the connection to stroke, we would NEVER have succumbed to allowing this so called "neck treatment" to be administered.

Because of this ongoing and updated wealth of information, there is a bright light heading towards the strange world of chiropractic; and it's not the Tooth Fairy. Can you say…FREIGHT TRAIN?!

༺༻

Sandy's Thoughts

I wish I knew then, what I know now.

Chapter Fourteen

∽⧚∾

Moving Forward

It was December 23, 2012; another typical cold winter day here in Edmonton.

We got back from Maui a few weeks ago. We had decided that Sandy was well enough to travel and I have mastered getting her in and out of washrooms very quickly.

The airplane trip was interesting, as they had to put us in the 19th row. For all those who had their wigs torn off and sleep disturbed while Sandy traversed the long isle, we sincerely apologize. To the Einstein who designed the washroom, I pray you will never have to go through what we did.

Still, despite the challenges of travel, it was wonderful to once again experience the joy this always brought to us.

We have adopted Maui. The people there are so friendly and were always very accommodating to Sandy's unique needs. On one occasion, just before heading up to see Haleakala's magnificent moonlike crater, Sandy advised me that she had to use the washroom. We had already been driving for the better part of the day having just explored the northern tip of the Island. (Definitely not for the faint of heart!)

Fortunately there was a rest area located in the state park that we had just passed. I turned the car around and headed back towards the entrance just before the last turn off.

Feeling really good about my keen sense of direction, and having caught a glimpse of the sign, I parked and got out of the car, assembled the wheelchair and we were off.

This shouldn't take long. As I pushed Sandy up the trail I discovered that the pavement ended. Oh well, just a long grassy stretch and we would be there. The goal was in clear site as we spotted the washroom facilities only about a hundred yards away.

Suddenly, about half way there, we began sinking. I tried turning around; but it just got worse. The sun was shining; but I was not happy at that moment. I pushed with all my might and we budged a few inches. I looked to my left and saw a woman sitting at a picnic table with her children. They were all watching this dumb tourist and probably wondering why we took this entrance. About 500 feet further down this road was a perfectly paved stretch of walkway complete with a parking area for the disabled. It led right to the facilities.

I decided to grunt it through and eventually we arrived at our destination, only to find a crowd of women each displaying a look of despair. Apparently the only other "stall" was not fit for any human to venture near. Subsequently, the line was long, and we thought we were in big trouble.

Were we to forgo the washroom break, we would never make it up the 10,000 foot rise in elevation with a full bladder. Fortunately, all but one of these kind ladies let us proceed to the front of the line. There would be no sneaking into this women's washroom. With no bag to place over my head, we proceeded forward.

This story would not be of particular worthiness to even mention were it not for the fact THAT SANDY DIDN'T HAVE TO GO! Try as she might, with the large audience pushed up against the door she experienced shy bladder syndrome. Despite my coaching and cheering her on, it was just no use.

We travelled back down the road until we found a public restaurant...and another restroom! Saved at last we enjoyed a great lunch and resumed our plans heading back up the sleeping volcano.

Despite Sandy's having a bit of a rough time with the altitude, once parked, she did agree to letting me push her up to the observation deck. She was not disappointed as we felt like we were on another planet. The views were incredible and beyond words.

While at the top, we watched a cyclist slowly climb his way to the summit. Some German tourists started clapping and we joined them in acknowledging his conquest. We couldn't believe our eyes. We estimated this fit man to be at least sixty-five years old.

One man asked him how long his journey had taken. "About five and a half hours from the base"; came his reply. I told him he must be in fantastic shape. He just looked at me and said, "No...just crazy."

I do not think Sandy will be doing this level of exercise anytime soon; but she has made me promise not to sell her bike. I wouldn't put anything past her, so like her golf clubs; I will keep it in storage...for now.

The time spent in Maui was a refreshing treat. Every day was a new adventure. We had missed so many years of enjoying the tropics, that we were determined not to waste a minute. Some of Sandy's fondest memories are of the putting green which was located directly below our condo's balcony.

Sandy would start her early mornings by sitting on the balcony with her Kona coffee and watch the daily ritual of golfers warming up for their game. She would laugh, sometimes a little too loudly, whenever there was a "pro" showing off his skills to his sweetheart. Often the highlight would inevitably come when the would-be student would sink her putts and leave her suitor in the dust. Sandy's sense of humor was showing again!

Another day we watched as a young, tanned bathing beauty, dressed in only a string bikini, practised her yoga on the same small practice area designated for the golfers.

One by one, the golfers left and the audience disappeared. I know what you are all thinking; BUT Sandy called *me* outside to see what was happening. Obviously Sandy is still very confident and knew I would see the humor in it. Still, a camera would have come in handy and the view would have made for quite the video…I mean for the exercise value, of course.

※

Sandy's Thoughts

Perhaps someday I will write a book solely based on our washroom experiences. Dave is a pretty smooth talker but as soon he discovers there are no family washrooms, he takes on a whole new personality, and his speed kicks into high gear. If I could figure out a way to motivate him to move this fast at home he wouldn't need to worry about his weight. There. I feel better now.

As for the bimbo on the putting green, well she's just lucky she couldn't hear me laughing.

I think that I should quit while I am ahead.

Chapter Fifteen

Sandy Gets the Last Word

David and I have been married for thirteen years. We fell in love almost immediately, although I had met David a few years prior to actual really dating him.

My family was leery of my getting involved with someone who had been previously married and also expressed deep concerns that he was much older than I was. In fact, David had been married twice before; so they were certainly warranted in their concerns.

However, with the passage of time, David won over their hearts as well and we eventually wed at a beautiful hotel located in heart of the Canadian Rockies. I will never forget the day we cemented our relationship, committed our love for each other and truly began our journey. I would never be alone again.

David had the respect of so many people. His business thrived probably due to the passion he had for his work. A "people person" with an outgoing friendly disposition, he had the best of clients. There are many, who, to this day still call and want him back in business. I was always proud of his accomplishments; but more so of what he stands for and the convictions he remains committed to this day.

I am so lucky to have a husband who cares so deeply for me. I would watch him as we went through those dark days and months together, during my long recovery, when he would negotiate on my behalf. David has a way with words. He was often gentle but firm and unwavering with the nurses and doctors. I truly worried for him the day he blocked the doorway to my hospital room while he waited for the security guards to remove him; but it showed me that he was willing to do whatever it took to protect my interests and well-being. He made me feel safe.

I really like this book; and feel it is an accurate assessment of how things were and how they are today. We continue to work together and hope to someday write another book. For now though, this has been enough for both of us.

It's interesting but I would often sit in our home office and just listen to David typing away. From time to time when reading something to me, and obviously reliving the moment, he would break down and start crying.

It was during this time that I have been able to provide comfort to my David. It's been an interesting switch of rolls after his having to always be the strong one…always the pillar. His guard is down; and I am once more able to reach out and hold him in my arms; or at times just encourage him to stop writing and get his wind back.

This stroke has been the trial of my life. Perhaps one of the worst things I had to experience was the constant suctioning of my throat. It deprived me of much sleep over an agonizing length of months. There was also the constant thought of whether or not this was to be my last day here on earth. I was at peace to leave but always felt my purpose here on earth was far from over.

In the past I had a lot of stress related issues; but just accepted that this was who I was. I would go on about things over and over, until those around me would go crazy. My nature had always been like this…until now.

Something happened during the recovery from my stroke that went beyond medical science. Something very positive! My being able to stand, despite the lingering balance issues, is wonderful. To have regained some of my abilities to speak and eat certain foods again, is beyond great; but for me to not have any more issues whatsoever with my stress controlling my life, is spectacular! I would compare it to a veil being lifted.

What were once becoming fears for me, and taking over my ability to enjoy even the simplest of life's pleasures, are now things of the past. I still have physical challenges; and life is different for me; but the mind is something that controls everything. You might as well not even have legs if you are too afraid to venture off the ship!

I am looking forward to what I hope will be my last surgery. The healing of my jaw continues to progress favorably. The plastic surgeon says this voice of mine should improve somewhat with my next surgery; however there are some risks involved. I will soon be going through another gambit of tests to determine if in fact this is still a viable option. We must tread carefully and weigh out all the possibilities as we have come so far. There is no way I want to take a step backwards!

David asked me what I wanted for this book to convey to others. I told him that I hoped it will ultimately make people think twice about having their necks twisted…by anyone, regardless of his or her title. Perhaps by having heard of my struggles and near brush with death, people will reconsider having an upper neck manipulation. I also hope that our story as a couple will help both men and women deal with the everyday stresses of life, and as a result of our relationship and its values, others also would come to realize how important it is to stick together through the good times and the bad. We all need each other.

My husband says that anyone in the medical field who has knowledge of these risks yet continues to practice this rapid upper neck twisting manoeuvre has blood on their hands. All they have to do is admit there are dangers that exceed any possible benefit and move on. Abolish this one single aspect and method of "treatment" and he will be a happy man. David is still very upset about what continues to go on within the chiropractic field in particular.

Perhaps more than anything, I recognize that there is coming a day when all of us will have to spend some time being looked after by others. Our bodies do break down as we age; illness occurs and accidents do happen. It's a part of living.

As sure as the sun comes up every morning, there will be challenges. My encouragement to all would be to hang in there and support those to whom you are committed and to rekindle your love today for each other; and build for the future hills and valleys that will surely come.

Life and death are certain for all of us. In fact, we recently opened an email from Stu and Laura, two of our angels, and very special cousins. They had sent us a quick note telling us they haven't forgotten about us. Then, like a brick falling out of the sky, shared the following information.

Stu's sister, his brother-in-law and mom were heading over to their place for lunch. The table was set and they were excited about seeing everyone. Not ten minutes away from arriving at their home in Spruce Grove, tragedy struck. Sadly, their mom died instantly at the scene, his brother-in-law and sister were also seriously injured in the crash. Sadly, the driver who lost control of her van also perished as a result of this accident.

We attended Stu's mother's funeral, and it was apparent by the large crowd in attendance, that she was truly loved!

We had watched the local news a few days prior; and like most things viewed on TV, you never think it's part of your life or connected with anyone you know. The carnage was awful; and now it hits close to home.

Stu's sister had been a primary caregiver and had lovingly attended to her mother over the years. Their mom was ninety-six years young; and had led a life of caring for everyone in need. But the hearts of many are hurting from their loss; and I was honoured to be able to attend and lend a shoulder. They have always been the ones comforting us. This was just one more reminder to us all, of the importance of living every day; because there are no guarantees in life. Just like with my past, everything can change in the blink of an eye.

I want to personally thank everyone for being a part of my life; for not giving up on me; and for believing in me...for believing in miracles. Thank you for drying my tears, brushing my hair, holding my hand and holding me tight; for encouraging me when the days grew dark; for standing up and giving me a voice when I could not be heard. Thank you, also, for making me not feel like a statue when you entered my room and engaged me in "conversation"; for helping David, my loving and devoted husband, make it through this nightmare and also survive his own ordeal.

I wish to thank all of the many nurses and doctors for all of the care, love and compassion they showed towards me in trying to understand and enter this world of silence and paralysis into which I had been thrown. It was a scary place.

Many thanks to those loving souls who took time out from their already busy schedules and organized the gala that provided so much aid at a time when we had financially reached rock bottom; and to the strangers, some of whom we had never even met, who came to our side and restored our faith in humankind. And of course for those who prayed around the clock for miracles. I felt the presence of a peace that went beyond all human understanding.

Despite the past, I want to make a difference in this world. I told David early during my hospital stay, that no matter what happened, and should I die...to please not let my death be without purpose.

I want so badly to help others and show them that they needn't carry the burdens all on their own. My faith was tested beyond measure; but never my belief that there was not a reason for everything that was happening.

Not everyone has the same support in place. I, too, saw the suffering of others while they sat all alone in their hospital rooms with no one to comfort them in their time of great need.

I am thankful for my faith in God. He gave me a good husband and supplied me with the inner strength when I could no longer move forward. He gave me purpose and direction. I feel sorry for those who travel similar roads alone when there is no need to do so.

I like the place I am today. I am not satisfied with where I am physically; but I am enjoying a peace within, that defies all logic. I love life. I love my family and friends. Any pain that others have caused me over the last five plus years is now forgiven and forgotten. Now the focus is to just keep pushing for the best my body will allow me to achieve; and not set the bar too high. Patience is something that has improved for me; but I have by no means mastered this part!

We will design a house in a few years that will provide me with a bit more independence; besides, David says he hates stairs and wants me to someday push him around in a wheelchair. He reminds me that he is ten years my senior and says this was the deal all along when he married me. I tell him, that unlike his, my mind is functioning just fine; and I have no recollection of that conversation.

I am starting to be able to help with dressing myself; so I've had to do a little more clothes shopping lately. We are getting ready for a cruise with some dear friends and I needed some outfits with a little more bling. You know...a girl's Gotta do what a girl's Gotta do!

Love and hugs,
Sandy

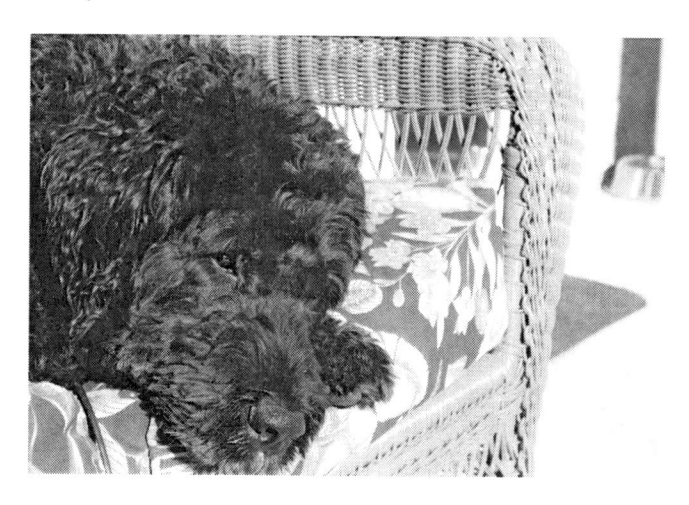

MICAH...MR. ATTITUDE

Update: We have a new addition to our family. Meet Micah everyone! He is a Bouvier de Flanders and at eighty five plus pounds his personality is as big as his mouth. His head is enormous and he gives Sandy the attention she so deserves. Now if I can just get him to quit trying to stop me from re-entering the bed during the night.

We rescued this fellow from the SPCA. It's hard to imagine anyone giving away this beautiful big guy. He is very protective, but not aggressive and already has bonded with Sandy. He looks like the little black Cockapoo we used to have... only on steroids.

Thank goodness I had him on a leash while out for one of our walks, because a buck and doe ran in front of us just a few feet away. Once my arms relocate I will write more about this breed.

Vacation Update 2013

We squeezed in one more vacation to escape the nasty cold grip of Old Man Winter. We both managed to snare a cold at the end of our cruise. Dave no sooner recovered when he was stricken with a serious bladder infection. The ambulance drivers were very kind and supplied my David with all the morphine he could handle.

Dave thinks the gal at the hospital might have been going through some kind of personal crisis, perhaps a nasty divorce. She told him to quit jumping off the gurney and spread his legs. Apparently my husband's enlarged prostrate gave her quite the challenge and the catheter was her means of revenge. Oh that David....always exaggerating. After not being able to pass anything for sixteen hours David said he was quite relieved, but highly embarrassed when following the procedure, he was instructed to "walk" to the nearby x-ray department. They wanted to make sure there was nothing else blocking the waterworks.

It got better. About six days after the catheter got removed, Dave twisted his knee and it popped completely out of joint. Not good. Once again we called the EMS. Fortunately as luck would have it, it was the same driver. (Did I mention Dave has NO PAIN TOLERANCE?) They administered several shots of morphine and in about an hour and a half had him loaded into the ambulance. This time it was off to a different hospital--the same one where I was initially taken following my stroke. Lots of flooding memories came back for Dave he explained later as they wheeled him to the exact same triage where I was treated five years ago.

Dave enjoyed the laughing gas and by the time he arrived at the hospital he was feeling somewhat better. They drugged him and sent him home the next day once everything got checked out and they confirmed that he had not broken anything.

Several days later Dave woke up and had no feeling on the right side of his face. His eyelid drooped; he had no taste and could not smile properly. It turned out that Dave has something called Bell's Palsy. Connie, Dave's sweet sister, told him that he is in good company as a number of "good looking" actors have also contracted this nerve disorder. Hmm....I joked that we can share my bibs and catch his drool. Well, I am sure this will not last, as Dave has begun recovering quite nicely. He's in the home stretch now; but I think it might be a while before we take another holiday! Guess I just have to take it easy on him.

Hopefully most of you will never have to experience, or come close to experiencing, the challenges that Sandy has had to face. We do, however, have a story to tell; and one that will hopefully go beyond just the injury itself. Today is a gift, the present, and it's here for each and every one of us.

While Sandy was in the hospital recovering, there would be many days that we would not know if she was going to survive; but there were never days when we wanted to give up. The desire to hang unto life itself was an incredible force; and one that Sandy harnessed from the start. We had too many dreams to fulfill as a couple. We had arrived at what we thought was the perfect place in life.

Sandy's prognosis indicates she can expect a shorter life span; but then again, many of these same experts said it would be unlikely that Sandy would ever speak or walk again.

I would not bet against her, my friends. Sandy said it best, when one night just before I was leaving the hospital, she spelled out the following; "Let's make tomorrow, today, Dave."

Tomorrow must be lived today; for we do not know what tomorrow will bring. Today is the present we all have. Get those hugs in, and don't spend time trying to save the pretty paper...rip it open and enjoy!

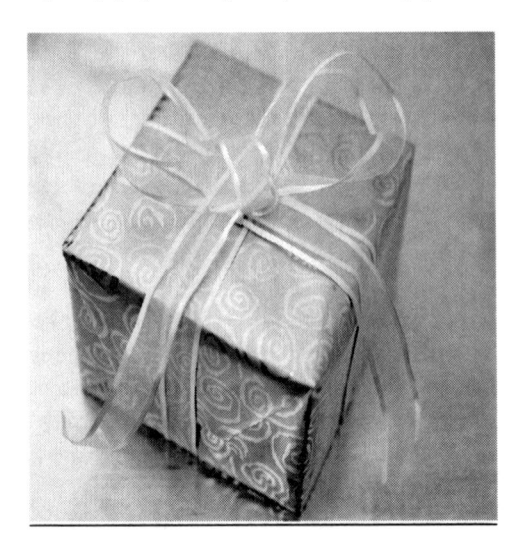